Birth Chairs,
Midwives,
and Medicine

Birth Chairs, Midwives, and Medicine

Amanda Carson Banks

University Press of Mississippi
Jackson

http://www.upress.state.ms.us

07 06 05 04 03 02 01 00 99   4 3 2 1
∞
Library of Congress Cataloging-in-Publication Data

Banks, Amanda Carson, 1965–
    Birth chairs, midwives, and medicine / Amanda Carson Banks
        p.   cm.
    Includes bibliographical references and index.
        ISBN 1-57806-171-7 (alk. paper). — ISBN 1-57806-172-5 (pbk. :
    alk. paper)
        1. Childbirth—Social aspects—History.   2. Midwifery—History.
    3. Birth customs—History.   4. Maternal health services—History.
    I. Title.
    RG652.B36   1999
    618.2'009—dc21   99-27105
                                                                    CIP

British Library Cataloging-in-Publication Data available

For September 9, 1983

If there be sermons in stones, there are surely volumes of romances in old furniture. And they are the best kind of romances, too, because they are all true and not the labored efforts of fictionaries, jaded with trying to find some new thing under the sun. We have but to open our eyes and unstop our ears to the language of furniture and a whole new world, richly filled with stirring memories, at once breaks upon us.

D. E. Eberlein and Abbot McClure,
The Practical Book of Period Furniture

Contents

Figures

Acknowledgments

Over the years, many people have played a part in seeing this book through to publication. I would like to extend my deepest thanks to three people who have had a primary role in this process: Craig Gill, my editor at the University Press of Mississippi, who has been continuously excited about this manuscript from its infancy as a dissertation and saw its potential even through the less-than-exciting conventions of dissertation writing; Robbie Davis-Floyd, my reader, whose words of wisdom, critical commentary, guidance, time, and support in reading and rereading the manuscript are unparalleled in kindness, thoroughness, and generosity; and David Hufford of the Pennsylvania State Medical College and the University of Pennsylvania, my dissertation committee chair and my advocate. There are not words to express my gratitude for all that you have done. Thank you.

I would also like to acknowledge friends and family who have been supportive in numerous ways. Significantly, I would like to thank Jeremy Teaford, my photographic consultant; Gaia Banks, my translation consultant; Melanie Lewis, who let me share in her pregnancies down to the most minute detail; Tanja Cutting, for duty above and beyond the call of friendship—reading the first draft; Tyrone Yarbourgh, who told me that if I wanted to know about birth chairs, I needed to write the book; Hal Dasinger, for his critical eye, editing pen, and so much more; and my family: Marjorie and Doug Nunn, for joining in the process and tracking down birth chairs; Helen Banks, for her rousing encouragement; and Diane, Gaia, Carrie, Hosanna, and Clare, for listening to me endlessly opine on the topic.

Finally, I would like to acknowledge the many curators and archivists of the European and American museums with whom I corresponded and did fieldwork: Gerhard Bott, Germanisches Nationalmuseum; David Nunn, London Hospital Medical College; Dieter Eisleb, Museum für Völkerkunde Berlin; Z. Gajda, Akademia Medyczna im. M. Kopernika in Krakowie; Juris Salaks, Paula Stradina Medicinas Vestures Muzejs-Riga; U. Tröhler, Georg-

August-Universität Göttingen; Heinrich Lakämper-Lührs, Stadtmuseum Gütersloh; Elfriede Priller, Oberösterreichisches Landmuseum; Janet Carding, National Museum of Science and Industry in London; Christine Speroni, Ville de Strasbourg; Christoph Mörgeli, Medizinhistorisches Institut und Museum der Universität Zürich; Manfred Skopec, Institut für Geschichte der Medizin der Universität Wien; Susan Case, Clendening History of Medicine Museum at the University of Kansas; Mona Kelly, Hemingway House Museum; Marcia Crandall, Cupola House Museum; Gretchen Woden, Mütter Museum of the College of Physicians of Philadelphia; Judy Chelnick, Smithsonian Institution; Nancy Evans, Winterthur Museum; and Barbara Poss, Terry Hambrecht, William Lyman, and Elizabeth Heathman. My thanks to you all and to all with whom I have spoken with over the years.

Introduction:
Artifacts and the Cultural Construction of Birth

In *Practica major,* Giovanni Savonarola (1384 –1461) described the common practices of childbirth and the predominant delivery methods of his day. "First then the midwife should prepare a stool on which to place the patient, and the patient may adapt herself in such a way that the birth may be made easy. The patient is placed in front of the semi circular part of the stool, and behind her is a woman who sits on the couch and holds her, and behind her, a little higher, is another against whom she leans, guiding and supporting herself."[1] In the midst of a medical lecture in 1947, however, Alexander Dempsey told of a very different origin of the birth chair.

Once there was a man, a carpenter by trade, living in Thuringia [Germany] at the beginning of the last century. This man gained such a reputation as an assistant at confinements from the fact that women sitting in his lap had a much easier delivery. He was, therefore, much in demand, and his calls to attend midwifery cases at all times were getting rather too much for him, so being of an inventive turn of mind, and a carpenter, he saw a way out, and invented and constructed our first-known aid to midwifery—the parturition [birth] chair.[2]

We have before us radically different accounts of the history of a fairly common artifact of birth and the historical way of birth. Although Dempsey's story is certainly colorful, it was only one of many similar versions presented in late-nineteenth-century and early-twentieth-century medical texts. The striking variation in accounts reveals that the history of birth chairs and, indeed, the general approach to birth has undergone radical reinterpretation and redefinition over time.

What can we infer from such differences in the history of birth and what do radical alterations in the practice of delivery indicate and reveal? Do such changes rest alone on developments in the knowledge and understanding of the physiology of birth and the development of medical expertise and technology to address this event? Or do such changes reflect shifts in the cultural meaning and significance attributed to birth and the associated structure of society as a whole? What is the history of birth from a material and a medical point of view? How intertwined should these perspectives be? Does one drive the other or are they independent?

Until fairly recently, the history of birth has been presented as a continuation of medical expertise and technology—charting *developments* not *changes* in the birth process. In the past, the texts concerning the history of birth (almost all written by doctors) reflected little of traditional attitudes. They were the descriptions of practices undertaken and advocated by the elite, the medical professionals. These texts did not capture or discuss the experiences of the vast majority of women giving birth nor did they address the attitudes or issues of contemporary society. Because these topics were glossed over in the past, they are all but unavailable to us now. After the medical community became more interested in childbirth, techniques became well documented, although textual accounts of the ideas, beliefs, and attitudes of women and society continue to be largely absent from literature written from the medical perspective.

No event, especially one as overlaid with cultural significance and popular wisdom as birth, can be technological alone, devoid of symbolic meaning and cultural significance. As a cultural construction, birth is intimately associated with the attitudes and beliefs that society holds toward the event—the values, needs, and perspectives of the community as a whole and the changing cultural context and societal significance and meaning of those involved. In fact, the way in which a society practices birth, the actual technical approach to delivery at any given time, is at root shaped by the way that a society interprets birth at that time. As Brigitte Jordan states in *Birth in Four Cultures,* "A society's way of conceptualizing birth constitutes the single most powerful indicator of the general shape of its birthing system . . . we find that whatever the local conceptualization of birth may be, that conceptualization powerfully directs the ways in which the physiology of parturition is socially interpreted in the collaborative, consensual doing of birth."[3]

Jordan offers a definition of birth in a biosocial framework, that is, "a phenomenon that is produced jointly and reflexively by (universal) biology and (particular) society."[4] In accomplishing this, Jordan presents a cross-cultural analysis of contemporary birth practices in Yucatan, Holland, Sweden, and the United States. She studies those features that encompass both the social and the physiological and medical aspects of the birth event to discuss and compare the universal biology of birth as it is mediated and interpreted by culture-specific practices.[5] Jordan does this through extensive anthropological fieldwork, analysis of practices and beliefs, and analysis of the artifacts of birth.

Likewise, developing a history of birth requires addressing the technical evolution of birth practices as *only a part of* the larger cultural construction of birth, including society's way of conceptualizing as well as its way of doing. It requires study of the practices of birth in relation to the history of the developing field of professional medicine, but it also fundamentally involves economics; traditional attitudes and beliefs about medicine, birth, and religion; a social understanding of women and their bodies; and the history of the society and culture as a whole. More recent works that address the social history of birth have accomplished a great deal in this area by uncovering and interpreting traditional practices and attitudes, but they are somewhat limited by the available documentation.

Stepping off from Jordan's analysis of birth in the twentieth century, I propose that we use a modified version of her biosocial framework and artifact approach to study the history of birth. Although we cannot perform anthropological fieldwork on the past or observe and interview midwives and parturients of past centuries, birth practices and their evolution can be studied through the material items that remain. Thus, the associated attitudes, beliefs, meanings, and understandings of birth that produced and drove these changes can be revealed because "a group's definition of the event becomes visible in its members' notions of what constitutes adequate justification for the practices in which they engage."[6] That is, a group's notions become visible through the artifacts it fabricates.

How can a material item created hundreds of years ago illuminate and describe? As Henry Glassie maintains, if we can comprehend people of the past through their material culture and through the artifact, the object that was a part if that material culture, we can create a more democratic history. His discussion of moving inward from the artifact to inspect the culture through the individual, instead of outward in a quest for hypothetical origins, is particularly important and useful in this study of birth. Glassie makes clear that any theory of history also requires a theory of culture, thereby allowing us "to conceive of individuals, their contexts, and their intentional actions as logical, systematic, interrelated and symbolic."[7]

This is not to say that a culture consciously records its ideas and attitudes in its material culture and that a maker of birth chairs is building with an intent to broadcast a message. Nevertheless, someone who makes a material artifact has a point of view regarding the artifact's purpose and value and implies an understanding of its immediate cultural context, intent, and style of use. As Jules Prown states, "objects made or modified by man reflect, consciously or unconsciously, directly or indirectly, the beliefs of the individuals who made, commissioned, purchased or used them and, by extension, the beliefs of the larger society to which they belonged."[8] In this way, a society's ideas, attitudes, and beliefs are imbedded in material artifacts. By corollary, items purposefully constructed for use during birth are emblematic of the prevailing philosophy and practices of birth—the cultural construction. Furthermore, because the practices of birth are a reflection of the current, prevailing attitudes of a society about birth, study of the popularity and use of birth artifacts; the subtle and overt alterations in their design, function, and use; and the changing textual accounts concerning them reveals cycles of emerging and prevailing, dated and fading ideas, attitudes, and beliefs of that society. Through the study of artifacts, we can regain and recreate a previously lost or vague area in the history of birth.

The field of material culture and artifact study, in general, and Jordan's discussion of the use of artifacts in understanding birth, in particular, become critical in developing a history of the cultural construction of birth. In fact, such study points to a gap in the scholarly literature about birth. Although the citizens of times passed have not left us a comprehensive social history or extensive writings detailing the perspective of the mother, the participants, or the community, they have left behind a large number of birth artifacts. A number of other scholars, such as Ann Oakley, Dorothy and Richard Wertz, Judith Walzer Leavitt, and Jane Donegan, have written excellent social histories of birth. None, however, have ever looked to the past to study what the artifact can tell us of the event, the process, and the belief. This is unfortunate because "the artifacts of birth, the objects and equipment . . . do more than deliver babies and cut cords: they are visible, practical constraints on which the shape of the system rests."[9] Specifically, as Jordan states, artifacts are "vehicles for gaining access to a specific way of doing birth; . . . they are available for observation, for asking questions of and about, and indeed, studying remarks and statements about them made by users and observers."[10] As a material, artifactual history of birth, a history of the birth chair can fill this gap. Where the texts are silent, material culture is eloquent.[11]

When studied in a social context, the artifacts of birth illuminate the cultural construction of birth—the system-specific definition of the birth process, a society's philosophy of birth, and the way in which the society enacts and practices the event. Analysis of the changing design and pattern of use of birth artifacts in association with social history, medical advancements, and attitudes about the participants make possible our identification of what attitudes and beliefs were active in the surrounding society, what needs and demands of society were present, what forces shaped and drove the way society constructed its understanding and defined the birth event, and most importantly, how such attitudes affected the way delivery was actually practiced.

To quote Jordan, "Methodologically, artifacts possess one nice quality that recommends them as vehicles for gaining access to a specific way of doing birth: in contrast to such intangibles as conceptualizations or expectations or attitudes, artifacts are visible and manipulable and thus directly available for the investigator's observations, for the asking of questions about them, for listening to talk regarding them, and sometimes, even, for gaining firsthand experience in using them."[12] Thus, a study of the material culture of birth allows us to tangibly see how the attitude toward and practices of birth have changed, even though we lack fieldwork, firsthand accounts, and documentary evidence. A material cultural analysis is complimented by or complimentary to the larger biosocial analysis. By studying material culture, we can understand how and why the definition and practices of birth experienced such a radical alteration, as evident in the quotations that began this introduction.

Although many artifacts of birth hold this telling information, the birth chair is particularly suited for a material reading of the story of birth. As we will see, birth chairs have a history characterized by varied and conflicting attitudes, interpretations, and stories; they have undergone telling alterations and innovations in design and use throughout their history; and they have more or less continued as a birth item until the present. It is not the birth chair alone that interests me, but rather what the birth chair, as an artifact, can tell us about actual practices and how these changed and developed.

It is the stories these chairs can tell of the altering and prevailing attitudes and beliefs—the driving philosophies of birth in the communities that designed, built, used, altered, and adapted them. Such a material analysis requires chronologically charting design and alterations in use and associating them with historical developments; attaching meaning to the alterations in design; focusing on the adaption to birth chairs that had proven adequate for years; looking at the innovations in design that coincide with the new requirements of current ideology; identifying movements that instigated changes in style, posture, and practice; and associating these changes with societal forces and developments. A material analysis requires placing the history of birth chairs within the larger societal context of birth and thereby helping to identify the influential changes in the prevailing philosophy of birth and the way in which these changes interacted with the material artifacts of the birth process.

A single chair, however, cannot tell the complete story, nor can a collection of chairs. Although birth chairs supply the focus for my discussion, it is in conjunction with associated materials and histories that they can reveal the pattern and process of the cultural construction of birth. Thus, I also consulted midwifery and obstetrical texts, artistic representations of birth, literary references to pregnancy and birth, historical accounts, and personal diaries for critical contextual information about societies' interpretations and understanding of birth and actual delivery practices. Together these items provide a means to discover and decipher the influence and effect of changing cultural ideologies and societal attitudes.

Birth Chairs as Social Indicators

Birth chairs are indeed interesting, but one may ask what revealed them to me as social indicators. Exodus 1:16 recounts Pharaoh telling the Hebrew midwives to watch for women who are "upon their stools." When I read this, I immediately asked myself, "What are these stools and what do they have to do with this passage and birth?" The discussions of the entomological issues of meaning and use in *Peake's Commentary on the Bible* (Black and Rowley 1997) were helpful, however, it was my brief reading of midwifery texts and ancient Near Eastern literature that first hinted to me that there was a much larger story at hand. Birth stools and birth chairs had a long, glorious history and then experienced a rapid fall from widespread popularity and use. Why? My fieldwork made it clear that birth chairs were not as obscure as one might imagine based on their place and mention in medical-historical works.[13] In fact, I found at least sixty birth chairs and stools dating from the 1600s through the 1900s on display in medical, anthropological, and ethnographic museums in Europe and North America as well as hundreds of antique and contemporary models in private homes, hospitals, birth centers, and with practicing midwives.

As I found more extant examples and located and identified more information about birth chairs, a pattern for birth chairs began to be revealed to me. Aesthetically, these chairs were certainly different and reflected culture, trends in style, and notions of design. There were also distinct changes and observable alterations in design from certain periods in history that could only reflect social changes. As the pattern began to emerge, I questioned what could have brought about these changes. I asked, "Why did birth chairs evolve as they did? Why did their design changes reflect more than developments in furniture design and style, more than advances in medical knowledge? And why did they all but disappear?" It is the attempt to answer such questions and the necessity to recapture a lost area of history that led to this material history.

Because this history rests in changing ideology and social contexts, it cannot linger in one period or geographical locale, but rather must encompass the cultural milieu of western Europe and North America over a period of hundreds of years and reflect the accumulation, interaction, and interrelationship of ideas. Specifically, I discuss how material culture can be used to observe changes in ideology and practice and how artifacts can be used to develop and flesh out an otherwise vague history. In this endeavor, I compare extant birth chairs dating from the eighteenth century well into the twentieth century and place them within their historical context. This time frame is not a haphazard choice or a mere reflection of the artifacts available. Rather, I chose this period because it is characterized by a drastic shift in the philosophy of birth and, therefore, the cultural construction of birth—a change so radical that an explanation must be sought. Birth chairs are critical in finding this explanation.

Birth was once regarded as a natural event calling for care within the community. However, by the late nineteenth century society changed its attitude toward birth to the extent that it came to be viewed as an inherently dangerous "disease state" requiring medical care and cure. The elements and practices associated with the earlier, more natural approach came to be regarded with apprehension and dread—representing a period before "treatment" was available, a time of the "dark ages" of medicine that lacked skill and expertise, a time of "meddlesome midwifery." By the turn of the twentieth century, birth had become the province of medical specialists who determined the process of delivery based on physiological understanding and their ideological requirements. As a medical specialty, birth required a set of associated techniques and proscriptions of practice. All interpretations of the history of birth were made to concur with the contemporary medical definition and practice of birth. In the late twentieth century, two diametrically opposed philosophies of birth, one represented by professional obstetrics and the other by the movement for alternative and/or natural birth, produced an era of combat for the control and the authority to define the prevailing philosophy and thereby shape the approach to delivery. In this period, as Jordan showed, it becomes obvious that the way a society or group approaches the birth event is predicated most clearly and significantly on how its members define birth and what they believe about it. As we will also see, this period reveals the utility of studying artifacts to develop a social history and the extent of the process of cultural construction, where ideology is reflected in artifact and where attitudes shape practice.

Therefore, the majority of the examples considered in this work range from the 1700s until the present, are of western European and North American construction, and are predominantly the material work of those of western European heritage. The artifacts, time frame, and geographical areas chosen for discussion were selected based on certain similarities of practice, ideology, medical advancement, and culture. Examples were also selected according to availability of artifacts to study and access to period texts; these were then refined to create a workable and comparable cross-section for study. Although there are significantly fewer American examples, this difference in number can be explained by the relatively shorter period of settlement prior to the explosion of changes in the field of obstetrics, the smaller number of medical schools and teaching hospitals (many Americans traveled to Europe in the eighteenth century for medical study), the few possessions carried by immigrants and settlers, and by a scarcity of scientific and ethnographic museums where these items could have been stored at the time they fell out of popularity.[14] I conducted additional research in European medical archives and ethnographic museums, making some prearranged visits and dropping by others and discovering birth chairs. Many items were haphazardly stored in archive warehouses, some were examined and measured in dark and dusty museum cases, and some I even took the opportunity to sit in while the curator went out for tea. I also corresponded with archivists; visited and interviewed a number of American midwives, directors of birth areas in hospitals and alternative birth centers, and mothers; and did additional fieldwork in Europe and America. Together, such fieldwork and research makes possible a more complete material history of the birth process.

Notes

1. Quoted in translation in Thompson (1921: 14).

2. See Dempsey (1949: 111). Gélis (1991: 289, n. 52) and Giron (1906–1907: 33) both offer versions of this story, but instead of a German, we have a Dutch carpenter. These narratives are also significant in that they provided a male genealogy for the origin of the birth chair.

3. Jordan (1993: 48–49).

4. Jordan (1993: 3).

5. Jordan (1993: 9).

6. Jordan (1993: 49).

7. Glassie (1988: 67). See also Glassie (1968).

8. Prown (1988: 18).

9. Jordan (1993: 87).

10. Jordan (1993: 81).

11. As Simon Bronner (1996: 463) states, "the special emphasis in material culture study is on the way that a material-environment is formed or cultural ideas and traditions are expressed in material form and construction activities."

12. Jordan (1993: 81).

13. Fieldwork included written inquires to anthropological and ethnographic museums of Europe, Great Britain, and the United States; archival research; and luck. As a graduate student, I arrived at the archive of the Thomas Jefferson University Hospital to discover that they had a birth chair on display.

14. The number of extant examples from Germanic areas supports this theory. In Germany, the rise of university-based midwifery programs and medical and science museums began early and often included the establishment of an archive or museum where such items were housed.

Birth Chairs,
Midwives,
and Medicine

Stones and Stools:
An Early History of Birth Chairs
and the Practice of Delivery

Long before delivery rooms, operating tables, stirrups, fetal monitors, and forceps, birth practices were simpler and less invasive. Women turned to other women, midwives (meaning literally "with women"), and practiced strikingly similar traditions of birth across time, place, culture, and geography. Birth was the province of women, with mothers, sisters, neighbors, and midwives striving together. Anthropological and archaeological evidence suggests an early confidence in the ability of women to bear children without intervention. For thousands of years the associated practices of birth were predicated on the apparent logic of merely assisting nature as it was allowed to take its course. Within the confines of nature, the mother controlled the process of the birth event.

Originally women gave birth kneeling or while sitting in an assistant's lap. In this posture, the women maintained a physiologically optimal, upright position without the interference of a bed, closed seat, or the ground. This style of delivery is implied in Genesis 30:3 when Rachel desires to have a surrogate child through her maid, "here is my maid Biliah; go into her that she may bear upon my knees, and even I may have children through her" (Figure 1.1).[1] Beyond the physiological effectiveness of such a manner of delivery, this approach strengthened the emotional bond between mother and assistant and built the connection between the community of women and their role in birth. The widespread use and the persistence over thousands of years of objects made to assist such a style of birthing indicates not only the prevalence and consistency of such practice and a confidence in the legitimacy and efficiency of such practices, but an associated philosophy of birth as a natural event.

The earlier fabricators or borrowers of objects made to assist in the

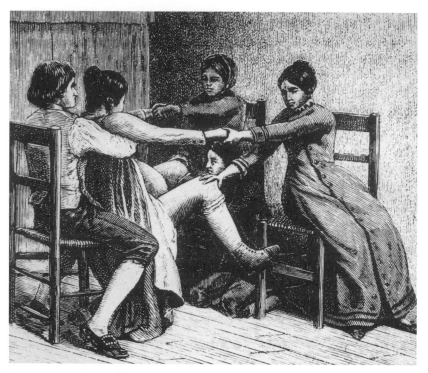

Figure 1.1. A variant of lap birth as depicted by George Engelmann in Labor among Primitive Peoples *(1882).*

birthing process clearly had this style of delivery in mind when they fashioned external items or altered existing objects. The first external, material objects used were birth stones and stools. Birth stones were two pieces of roughly shaped rock placed slightly apart so as to create a makeshift seat or stool with an opening in the middle on which the mother sat or kneeled.[2] In fact, the Egyptian hieroglyphic for birth was rendered as a woman giving birth while seated on two stones.[3] Such a "stool" supported the mother's bottom above the ground, and an assistant held her about the waist for balance. This may explain the confusion over the translation of the Hebrew word "Elhabim," which is given alternately as "stones" or "stools" in Exodus 1:16. Although the Bible's value as a historical source continues to be debated, it is accepted as a source of cultural information. This passage in Exodus reflects the use of fabricated birth items as early as the period reliably fixed at 1400 B.C.E.[4]

Squatting, sitting in the lap of an assistant, and the use of stones were eventually replaced by more permanent birth stools, which became the predominant item fabricated for use in delivery in most cultures. Early use of birth stools is indicated by several sources, for example, a depiction of an Egyptian queen giving birth on a stool appears on the walls of the Birth House at Luxor, Egypt (c. 1450 B.C.E.); a sculpted votive from ancient Greece (c. 200 B.C.E.) showing a woman using a tripod birth stool; and a bas-relief from the Roman period (c. 200 C.E.) of a woman seated upon a birth stool or chair while three women display her newborn child. Clearly, fabricated objects to assist birth were so closely associated with the birth process in the popular mind that when a first-century Roman artist wanted to depict the birth of Athena from Zeus's head, he placed Zeus on a birth chair (Figure 1.2).[5]

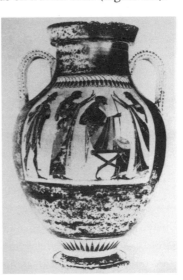

Figure 1.2. Roman amphora from Italy, c. first century C.E. Seated on a birth stool, Zeus prepares to give birth to Athena. He is attended by the Eileithyiai, the Roman goddesses of childbirth. From Harold Speert, Incognita Gyniatrica *(1973). Reprinted by permission.*

The use of birth stools was not isolated in space and time to the ancient world, however. Votive offerings from wells active in the Celtic period (c. 100 C.E.) in Britain portray women giving birth in sitting or squatting postures, possibly on fabricated items, and anthropological evidence relating to early non-European cultures reveals the use of a variety of upright birth postures assisted by fabricated items.[6] Worldwide examples are plentiful, as seen in artwork and as recorded in missionary chronicles of culture and society in Asia and as supported by anthropologists studying Africans, nomadic cultures of the Near East, South Pacific Islanders, and early historians writing about Native Americans (Figure 1.3).[7]

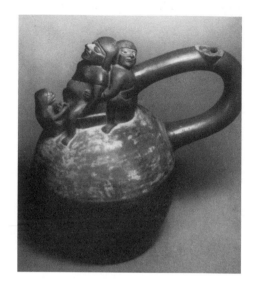

Figure 1.3. This pre-Columbian vase from Peru depicts a midwife delivering a child while the mother sits upon a birth stool and is supported from behind by an assistant. Photograph courtesy of the Museum für Volkerkunde Staaliche, Berlin.

In fact, due to their prominence, birth chairs came to signify birth so completely that artists and authors merely had to introduce the birth stool or chair to convey the idea of delivery. To recount the story of the birth of Jacob and Esau, a woodcut from a Passover Haggadah from fourteenth-century Sarajevo placed Rebecca on a birth chair. A simple birth scene from a 1497 edition of Ovid's *Metamorphoseos Vulgare* depicts the birth of Hercules with Alcmena comforted by three attendants as she sits on a birth chair with a midwife before her.[8] In his play *The Magnetic Lady* (1640), Ben Jonson named his characters by their profession; along with Compass the mathematician, Captain Ironside the soldier, Practice the lawyer, and Needle the tailor, Jonson wrote about Mistress Chair, the midwife. When Needle brings her to a delivery, Mistress Chair states:

> *Stay, Master Needle, you do prick too fast,*
> *Upon this business I must take some breath;*
> *Lend me my stool;*
> *You have drawn a stitch upon me,*
> *In faith, Sir Needle, with your haste.*[9]

As the needle was the tailor's tool, so the midwife's was a birthing stool.

In the days when people considered birth a normal process of nature, they were content to allow nature to follow its course. The predominant practices, associated material items, and, indeed, the very language were predicated upon this philosophy of birth.[10] The *Encyclopaedia Britannica* (1771) reflected such a philosophy by defining midwifery as "the art of *assisting* nature in bringing forth a perfect foetus, or child from the womb of the mother" (emphasis added).[11] Intervention was rare and was usually undertaken only in the case of an impossible delivery or the death or near death of the mother or child in utero. Doctors were called only in dire situations. Society regarded midwives and women of the community as sufficient and capable attendants, and these women enjoyed high community status. The practices of delivery and the material artifacts of birth reflect this as well. Birth stools were simple, noninterventionist, and merely assisted nature as it took its course.

The Design of Birth Chairs

Pictorial descriptions and extant examples of birth stools from the later Middle Ages are fairly numerous. The designs, which were possibly directed by the local midwives, reflected regional ideas of furniture construction, traditions of birth lore, and aesthetic notions. These stools were devices shaped to ideally perform their function rather than to decorate, following the dictum "form follows function." Birth stools merely assisted or mimicked the physiological natural, upright posture.[12] Designs were unregimented, as was the general practice of delivery. Some stools were very rudimentary; some were obvious adaptations of already available standard chairs; some were practically without ornamentation, whereas others were quite specialized with decorations, engraving, and personalization. Although countless innovations and differences are apparent from chair to chair and from community to community, birth chairs fabricated and used until the mid-1700s all served simply to assist the mother in birth, an event practiced "close to nature."[13]

Although birth stools were built in accordance with each community's or midwife's individual opinions and reflected their general matter-of-fact approach to delivery, the stools' general similarity resulted from the basic functional needs of the mother. They provided balance and support to assist the mother in the process of delivery. They accomplished this in various ways. Birth stools had three legs and possessed either a horseshoe-shaped opening in the seat or a very narrow, solid, rectangular seat about ten inches above the ground. Both styles supported the bottom of the delivering woman. Some had a sloping back with hand-holds fashioned on the edges of the seat or horizontal slats connecting the legs that produced a "Y" shaped opening about eight to ten inches from the ground. Birth chairs had four legs and a seat with the distinctively cut horseshoe or semicircular opening and a straighter back. All were designed to allow the laboring woman to sit rather than to support herself in a squatting position (Figure 1.4). The height of the seat on both stools and chairs made it possible for the delivering woman to brace her feet against the ground during contractions while still allowing attendants to have access to the birth canal. The limited back area also permitted attendants access and room to support and massage the mother's stomach. The hand-holds on many provided the mother with extra leverage to grip, push, and pull during contractions.

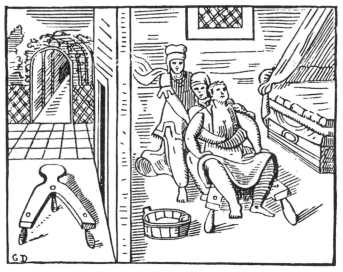

Figure 1.4. The style of a "Y" stool is clearly seen in this sketch taken from Giovanni Savonarola's Practica major, *first published in the fifteenth century.*

These items were often owned by a midwife, who brought them along when called to a delivery, as Jonson's Mistress Chair. A diary account by Samuel Sewall of Massachusetts portrays such a trip by a midwife: "April 2, 1677. Father and I sitting in the great Hall, heard the child cry . . . Went home with the Midwife about 2 o'clock, carrying her Stool, whose

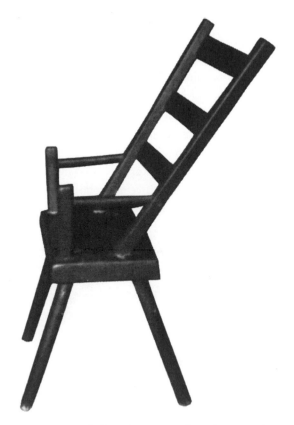

Figure 1.5. Birth chair, American, c. late 1600s or early 1700s. It is made of painted yellow pine or cypress. The chair is 37 inches high, 17.75 inches wide, and 11.5 deep. The solid seat is very narrow (10.5 inches wide) and is 15.5 inches above the ground. In the collection of the Cupola House, Edenton, North Carolina, the home of a doctor and his descendants for 141 years. The chair is assumed to have been one of his possessions that remained in the house from generation to generation. Photograph courtesy of William Lyman.

parts were included in a Bagg. Met with the watch at Mr. Rocks Brew house, who baid us stand, enquired what we were. I told the Woman's occupation, so they baid God bless our labours, and let us pass."[14] In some instances, the midwife of a region was recognized for her service and provided with a chair or a stool. For example, an account from the 1427 records of Stadt Baden in Switzerland notes that a midwife was hired to serve the town and in 1429 a "kindbetterstul," a birth stool, was purchased for her use.[15]

Popular, functional, and almost universal in basic design, birth stools and chairs of these styles continued to be built and used by midwives and non-medical personnel for hundreds of years. Throughout the time period covered by this book, their use was often in direct contradiction to the recommended, medically advocated changes in birth-chair design and the philosophy of birth. For example, sketches of such designs in manuscripts date almost exclusively to the seventeenth century, however, there were similar examples built and used in eighteenth-century America and nineteenth-century Spain (Figures 1.5 and 1.6).

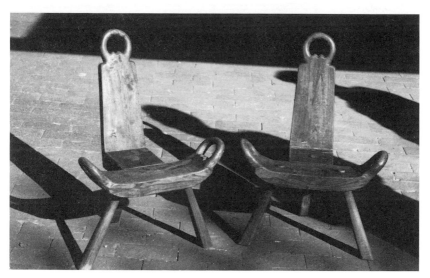

Figure 1.6. Birth stools, Spanish, c. 1800s, in the collection of the Museum of Pharmacy and Medicine, Tucson, Arizona. Purchased by the owner in Madrid, Spain, in 1963. The stools are approximately twenty-seven inches high. Hand-holds are shaped at either end of the narrow bench seats, which are approximately eleven inches above the ground. Photograph courtesy of Marjorie and Doug Nunn.

Apparently, the only texts discussing midwifery practices or depicting birth stools that were available during the early Middle Ages were translations or copies of earlier Greek and Latin texts by such people as Hippocrates, Soranus, and Galen. Those who studied medicine regarded these texts as sufficient for all knowledge. Because religious beliefs and laws—such as the purity laws in

Leviticus 15 and 20 and various papal edicts—discouraged and often outlawed any dissection or examination of the human body, there was little development of new knowledge of general medicine and internal anatomy.[16] As W. H. Williams later stated about this period, "So dazzled were the medical world with the splendid genius of Hippocrates; so confused and paralyzed by the contemplation of his astonishing industry; . . . that for 500 years they knelt at his shrine, and placed their highest merit in an undeviating imitation of his practice, and an implicit faith in his precepts."[17] Even as late as 1742, knowledge of the works of Hippocrates and Galen were regarded as all that was necessary to make a good doctor. For example, Henry Fielding's satire *Joseph Andrews* (1742) made reference to this:

"Books!" cries the doctor. "What, I suppose you have had Galen and Hippocrates!" . . . "Sir," cries the other, "I believe there are many surgeons who have never read these authors." "I believe so too," says the doctor, "more shame for them: but thanks to my education: I have them by heart, and very seldom go without them both in my pocket." "They are pretty large books," said the gentleman. "Aye," said the doctor, "I believe I know how large they are better than you," (at which he fell a winking, and the whole company burst into a laugh).[18]

With limited documentary evidence that can illuminate the social history, what we know of birth from earlier periods is largely drawn from artistic representations, brief textual references unrelated to midwifery, and the earliest midwifery texts. Although little was written about birth specifically and no known examples of birth chairs remain from before the 1600s, the sketches and artistic representations of birth support this interpretation of birth as simple. In these renditions, midwives and any number of female attendants are present and the chairs from the period appear simple in form.[19]

The chairs pictured in such artistic contexts, those described and sketched, and the later American and Spanish birth chairs in Figures 1.5 and 1.6 indicate that these styles of birth chairs remained fairly consistent over hundreds of years. The lack of detailed textual references to birth and the simple designs of birth chairs portray a view of birth as natural and unexceptional and labor and delivery as practical and efficient.

Birth Chairs in Early Midwifery Texts

European texts concerning midwifery and birth began appearing in the early sixteenth century and recounted simple practices of delivery that clearly

advocated a natural philosophy of birth. These texts were particularly important for the history of birth. Written not in Latin, like the works of
Hippocrates, Magnus, and Savonarola, but in the vernacular, such texts were
accessible to a larger audience than were the earliest texts and the oral
accounts of midwives. In addition, Gutenberg's invention of movable type
allowed the mass production of books, which thus strikingly increased the
availability of these texts. No account of a normal labor in these early midwifery texts advocated any interventions. Only in the cases of an impeded
birth or the presence of a dead infant were any specific interventions noted.
None fails to recommend the upright delivery; all advocate the use of a birth
stool or chair for assistance, in simple, direct language.

One of the first of these European books on midwifery was Ortloff von
Bayerland's *Das Frauenbuchlein* ("Little Book for Women," 1500). Besides
recommending an upright delivery position assisted by a birth stool, Ortloff
offered little detail about the process of delivery other than directing that the
process move toward its natural conclusion. Eucharius Rösslin, the city
physician of Frankfurt-am-Main, soon followed with a similar book, *Der
Swangern frauen und Hebammen Rosengarten* ("A Garden of Roses for Pregnant
Women and Midwives," 1513). This text was illustrated with woodcuts of
birth stools and midwives by Martin Caldenbach (?1470–1520), a student of
Albrect Dürer (1471–1528). Like Ortloff and others to follow, Rösslin
directed his text to practicing and knowledgeable midwives. Rösslin's son
translated the *Rosengarten* into Latin in 1532 as *De Tartu Hominis* and
Latinized his father's name to Rhodion. Although it was the same text, the
Latin version was something of a scholar's edition and was intended for doctors. The text was published in French as *Des divers travaulz et enfantemes des
femme,* and Dutch and Spanish editions soon followed. By 1540, Richard
Jonas translated Rösslin's work from the Latin into English as *The Byrth of
Mankynde.*[20] Thomas Raynalde published a second English edition in 1545,
enlarging the title to *The Byrth of Mankynde, Otherwyse Named the Woman's
Booke.* This text became a mainstay of English midwifery for the next hundred years. Raynalde's translation of Rösslin's text provides a description of
normal delivery:

Then it will be meet for her to sit down leaning backward (in the birth stool) in
manner upright. For the which purpose in some regions (as in France and Germany)
the midwives have stools for the purpose, which being not low, and not high from

the ground be made so round wise and concave or hollow in the middle, that they may be received from underneath which is looked for [the baby] and the back of the stool leaning backward received the back of the woman, the fashion of which the stool, is set in the beginning of the birth figures hereafter. And when the time of labor is come, in the same stool ought to be put many clothes or rags in the back of it, that which the midwife may remove from one side to another according as necessity shall require. The midwife herself shall sit before the laboring woman and shall diligently observe and wait, how much, and after what means the child stireth itself, also shall with her hands first anointed with the oil of almonds, or the oil of white lilies.[21]

Over the next hundred years Rösslin's work alone emerged in thirteen English editions and countless other German, French, and Spanish translations as well.[22]

The text of Jakob Rueff (1500–1558), Director of Midwives in Zurich, *Ein schon lustig Trostbuchle in von den Empfangnissen und Geburten der Menschen* ("Cheerful, Gay, and Comforting Little Book about the Conception and Birth of People," 1544) also described the practice and artifacts of birth and the basic tenor of societal attitudes toward the process. He briefly depicted the process of birth, dwelling on examples of the birth of "monsters." He suggested some tools, primarily crochets for dissecting a blocked or dead infant in utero, and described the attributes of a model midwife. Rueff also provided one of the clearer and more detailed accounts of delivery and the use of a birth stool of the time. Like Rösslin's text, Rueff's was also translated, first into Latin as *De Conceptu et Generatione Hominis* (1554) and then into English as *A Very Cheerful Book* (1559).

Such texts acknowledged midwives' skills and understanding of the event, thus indicating that women, both as midwives and as parturients, were considered capable of dealing with labor and delivery. For example, Ortloff apologized for leaving anything out, but assumed that midwives would notice his omissions: "And that is why, [my] dear women, after having been asked by you to write something for pregnant women, I beg you not to take offense if I have been too crude. Never was this my intention."[23] Rösslin instructed the midwife to "direct everything as shall seem best"; and Nicholas Culpepper, in *A Directory for Midwives* (1671), wished midwives "success in their Office in this World, and a Crown of Glory in that to come."[24]

Of course, that Ortloff, an Austrian, Rösslin, a German, and Rueff, a Dutchman, produced similar accounts does not prove that the general prac-

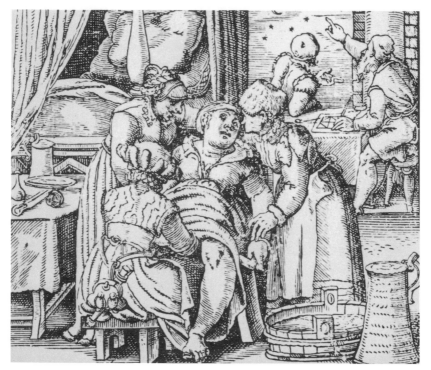

Figure 1.7. Woodcut by Jost Amman in Jakob Rueff's du Conceptu et generatione hominis *(1580). While a midwife attends to a woman seated on a birth chair, an astrologer charts the newborn's fortunes.*

tices of birth or the philosophy of birth as a natural event were universal throughout England and Europe. The proof is that similar texts offering the same advice and reflecting the same philosophy were written throughout Europe, there was a market for the translations of these texts, and mention and depictions of birth portray it as a natural event. This indicates that society, even the society of physicians, regarded birth as largely a process of nature to be observed, assisted, and best attended to by those close to the laboring woman.[25]

Artifacts and Philosophy

Birth chairs from the sixteenth and seventeenth centuries reflect this approach and support this interpretation as well. They were simple, uninvolved devices that merely offered support in an upright posture and were

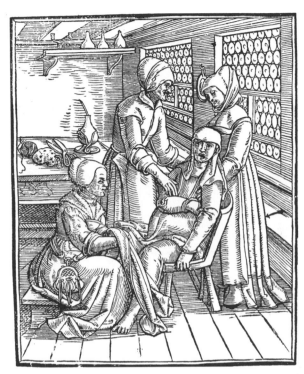

Figure 1.8. Woodcut, c. 1500s, from Jacobus Rueff's Ein schön lustig Trostbuchle von den Empfengknuben *(1554).*

used in delivery as a matter of course. We see this matter-of-fact attitude toward the event in artistic renditions of births and birth chairs from the period and in extant examples.

A woodcut from Jakob Rueff's *du Conceptu et generatione hominis* (1554) shows an astrologer charting the child's fortunes as the midwife is still assisting a woman seated on a birth stool. The 1545 edition of Rösslin's *Rosengarten* depicts a woman laboring while others dine and children play. Finally, a woodcut from Rueff's 1554 edition of *Ein schön lustig Trostbuchle* displays the typical, simple articles associated with midwives resting on the table: the ball of twine and the scissors, with the birth chair nearby (Figures 1.7 and 1.8). As Laurel Ulrich states regarding the work of eighteenth-century midwife Martha Ballard, "For many women, the first stage of labor probably took on something of the character of a party. One of the mother's responsibilities was to provide refreshments for her attendants. The very names *groaning beer* and *groaning cakes* suggest that at least some of this food

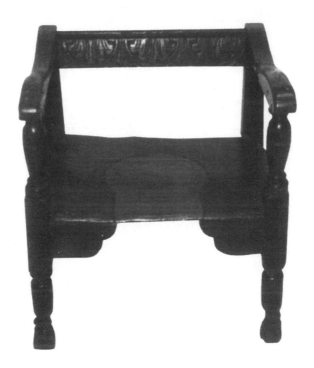

Figure 1.9. Birth chair, English, c. 1600s, in the collection of The National Museum of Science and Industry, London. Constructed of elm and oak, the chair is 26.25 inches high, 23.5 inches wide, and 20.5 inches deep. The seat is 12 inches above the ground and has a removable keyhole section in the seat. The opening appears to be a later addition due to its much cruder workmanship. The seat, back, and arms are fixed and feature a carved leaf motif. The front legs are baluster turned, are in better condition than the rest of chair, and are thus most likely replacements. Photograph by author.

was consumed during labor itself."[26] In these diverse examples, birth was an event that involved the community, included any number of helpers, and was practiced as a part of life, which continued as the birth proceeded.

Although this prevailing philosophy of birth was relatively consistent in western Europe, birth chairs' design and construction varied according to locale, carpenter, and midwife, while holding constant the essential form.

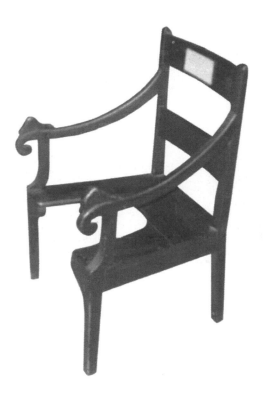

*Figure 1.10. Birth chair, Portuguese, c. early 1700s, in the collection of
The London Hospital Medical College, University of London. The chair is
33.25 inches high, 17.25 inches wide, and 20 inches deep. The seat is
13.75 above the ground. The back, seat, and arms are fixed, and the chair
does not fold for transportation. The college museum provides the following
text concerning the chair: "Its use in labour was verified by a Portuguese
doctor, who says they are still in vogue in the smaller villages. The patient,
seated in the chair, was comforted by her friends, while the midwife performed the necessary duties below. This chair was brought in a rummage
market in Lisbon, and is now exhibited by the owner, Mr. C. J. Tabor,
Knotts Green, Leyton, Essex (1802)." Photograph by author.*

Thus birth chairs changed in appearance, but in function and use they
remained simply fabricated items designed to assist nature in delivery.
Evidence of this is apparent through the examination of the earliest extant
birth chairs, which date from the seventeenth century. A classic example is
an English chair now owned by the National Museum of Science and

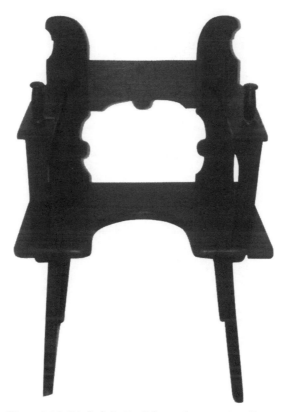

*Figure 1.11. Birth chair, English, c. 1600s, in the collection
of The National Museum of Science and Industry, London.
The chair is made of pine, and is 41.25 inches high, 20.75
inches wide, and 27.75 deep. The seat is 13 inches above the
ground. The back, seat, and hand-holds are fixed, and the
chair does not fold for transportation. The hand-holds are
made of different wood and are probably replacements.
Photograph by author.*

Industry in London. This English chair from the mid-1600s has open arms, separate legs, and an open back with a carved leaf motif running along the back slat and legs. Very telling is the semicircular seat opening with a removable keyhole section. Roughly hewn, this example was most likely converted into a birth chair because the workmanship of the seat opening is much cruder than the rest of the chair. This adaptation of an already existing chair indicates the absence of rigid conventions in birth-chair design and

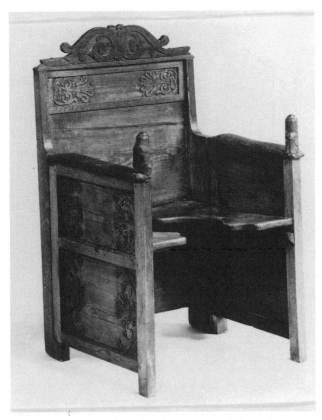

Figure 1.12. Folding birth chair, German, c. 1650, in the collection of the Germanisches Nationalmuseum in Nürnberg. Handsawn ornaments of pine are on the top and external sides, and the hand-holds and arms are covered in leather. The chair is 36 inches high, 20.5 inches wide, and 22 inches deep. The seat is 16 inches above the ground. The back and hand-holds are fixed, whereas the seat folds up and the sides fold in for easy transportation. Photograph courtesy of the Germanisches Nationalmuseum, Nürnberg.

approaches to the process of delivery (Figure 1.9).[27] Another example reflecting this simplicity is a Portuguese birth chair dating from the early 1700s (Figure 1.10). The chair is thirty-three inches high at its back, seventeen inches wide, and has a seat thirteen inches above the ground. The back, seat, and arms are fixed; it does not fold for transportation, although it is obviously small and lightweight.

Although all the extant chairs of this period have the characteristic semicircular seat opening at the optimal height of ten to thirteen inches above the ground, which was recommended by Rueff, the design, craftsmanship, and decorative aspects indicate individual, unique, and localized construction. An example that reveals this is an English birth chair from c. 1600–1650, also owned by the National Museum of Science and Industry (Figure 1.11.) While incorporating innovations in furniture design, the chair maintains the optimal seat height, semicircular opening, and hand-holds of earlier birth stools and chairs. The pine chair has open arms and back and separate legs and does not fold for transport.

Another style that is similar in function is a German birth chair of the same period (Figure 1.12). It is simple in design and bears the familiar semicircular seat opening, height, and hand-holds. However, this chair also exhibits local design styles, innovations like handsawn ornamentation on its back, and the popular panel style of seventeenth-century Germany. Now located at Germanisches Nationalmuseum in Nürnberg, this chair was constructed with a circular opening in the back, an innovation that allowed attendants access to the laboring mother for massage and support that the more substantial back might have precluded. This chair was also designed to fold for transport.

Similar, yet more original in design, is an American birth chair of a slightly later period (c. 1700–1750) that is owned by the National Museum of Science and Industry (Figure 1.13). Constructed of elm and beech in the Windsor style, this chair is lightweight, but did not disassemble for carrying or storage. Although probably altered to function as a birth chair, the prevailing characteristic of the seat design (the semicircular opening) and the simplicity of intent make this chair consistent with its continental cousins.

The available histories of birth that discuss birth chairs maintain that during the seventeenth and eighteenth centuries the use of stools and chairs was primarily restricted to urban women, whereas their rural counterparts retained the manner of standing or squatting. While providing numerous "exceptions" to this, historians justify this belief based on the infrequent mention of birth chairs in contemporary academic texts. However, these texts were accounts written in cities about events in cities, and they were chiefly concerned with the more decorative examples of birth chairs from the period.[28] These histories fail to consider that the birth practices of a rural population would likely not appear in writing because of lower literacy rates and the community's isolation from centers of learning and from those city physicians

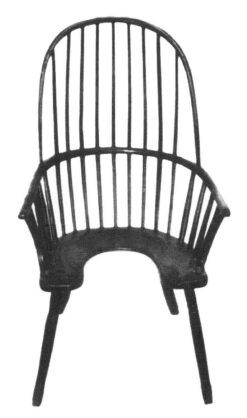

Figure 1.13. Birth chair, American, c. 1750–1760, in the collection of The National Museum of Science and Industry, London. This Windsor-style chair is constructed of elm and beech. The chair is 40 inches high, 22.5 inches wide, and 30.25 inches deep. The seat is 13 inches above the ground. The seat, arms, and back are fixed, and the chair does not fold for transportation. Photograph by author.

who were writing the midwifery texts of the day. Certainly, the artifacts of the urban and wealthy are much more likely to survive than artifacts of poor or rural people.[29] Such histories were correct in noting that the majority of the remaining birth chairs were the property of the urban wealthy. However, numerous accounts of birth chairs within local tradition and artistic renditions and the sheer number of birth chairs that do remain suggest a more widespread use of these chairs, many examples of which have not survived.[30]

The descriptions of the process of birth in midwifery texts began to be more detailed and anecdotal as time passed and more women were observed. For example, Louise Bourgeois (1563–1636), a practicing midwife at the Hotel Dieu in Paris, went beyond depicting birth posture and recounting earlier texts and offered anecdotal information based on her own experience. In *Les Six Couches de Marie de Médicis,* Bourgeois described how Marie de Médicis delivered on a red velvet birth chair in a special green-walled room with King Henry IV in attendance.[31] Bourgeois's attention to detail appears in her discussion of the variety of positions women chose for birth: standing, squatting, sitting, or on all fours. However, she advocated the use of birth chairs, except in cases of difficulty: "A woman who wishes to keep about and can do so until she is just ready to give birth to the child, may be allowed to stand with her legs apart, supported during the pains by two strong people, or she can have a low stool with a pillow on it, in front of a table, and can kneel on the pillow and put her arms on the table."[32]

The publication of midwifery manuals like those of Rueff, Rösslin, and Bourgeois attest to the common notion of a natural, noninterventionist approach to delivery through the birth scenes they depict and the labors and postures they describe. These texts also discuss the widespread use of birth chairs with midwives occupying a revered position, serving the community, the government, and the church.[33]

Societal Shifts, the Church, and Midwifery

The increase in the publication and dissemination of midwifery texts also reveals the buildup of underlying societal forces that eventually would have a great impact on the philosophy and the practice of birth. For example, during the Inquisition midwives were suspected of being witches.[34] Midwives also suffered social culpability when delivering a damaged or deformed child; later church regulations regarding midwives began to damage societal regard for midwives and their skills, and by association the role of women in birth.[35] Although the influence of the church lessened, such charges permanently affected the reputation of midwifery. Society began to question the need for midwives and even to suspect them of incompetence, evil, and squalor. Likewise, the gradually changing tone of midwifery texts, which became more directional and instructive, began to cultivate a different attitude and approach to midwives and, by association, women. This social atmosphere toward women characterized the beginning of the rise of profes-

sional medicine, when physicians wrote midwifery texts to educate practicing midwives as well as to regulate and control them.

Central to these changes in the atmosphere of birth, the practice of delivery, and the alterations in birth-chair design was the waning authority of the
Catholic Church and the release of medical study and inquiry from its constraints. For centuries the church had forbidden examination of the human
corpse and even, in many areas, the study of medicine. As the church's influence declined during in the Enlightenment, medicine was freed from the
outdated notions of Galen and other ancient writers and the confines of religious orthodoxy regarding sickness and health. This allowed new information about anatomy to be discovered and to infiltrate academic institutions
and for the eventual change in the gender of the practitioner. Significantly,
the establishment of facilities organized and run by governmental authorities and staffed by male physicians provided study material and case examples. At such centers, midwives attended all normal deliveries, but physicians often observed and began to assist at difficult or abnormal births. For
the first time, male physicians had the opportunity to consistently view
deliveries and to formulate ideas about the progress of pregnancy and the
process of delivery. The trend toward professional medical involvement in
birth had begun, along with a shift in the gender of the birth practitioner
from female to male.

Although the sixteenth and seventeenth centuries were characterized by
many changes in the understanding of birth, the publication of more detailed
midwifery texts, and the incremental development of forces that would eventually make a significant difference, there was at first little alteration in the
general community's perception and practice of birth. Although knowledge
had increased, societal issues that could apply enough influence to effect a
change in the philosophy of birth and, therefore, the general practice of delivery had not yet come to the fore. Even William Smellie (1697–1763), who
sought a more medicalized and professional obstetrical approach to birth,
acknowledged varying styles and practices without condemnation:

Among the Egyptians, Grecians, and Romans, the woman was placed on a stool; in
Germany and Holland, they use the chair which is described by Deventer and Heister, and for hot climates the stool is perfectly well adapted; but in northern
countries, and cold weather, such a position must endanger the patient's health. In
the West Indies and some parts of Britain, the woman is seated on a stool made in
the form of a semicircle: in other places she is placed on a woman's lap; and some,

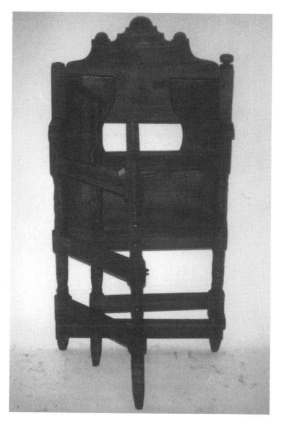

*Figure 1.14. Folding birth chair, European, c.
1750–1800, in the collection of The National Museum of
Science and Industry, London. The chair has walnut and
iron hinges and lathe-turned legs. The chair is 41.5 inches
high, 27.25 inches wide, and 21.25 inches deep. The seat
is 17 inches above the ground. The seat folds upward and
the sides fold inward for transportation. The seat engages
via two iron pins and eyes with sides when folded down.
Photograph by author.*

kneeling on a large cushion, are delivered backwards. In France, the position is
chiefly that of half-sitting, half-lying, on the side or end of a bed; or the woman,
being in naked bed, is raised up with pillows or a bed-chair.[36]

While descriptions from such texts as Smellie's indicate a growing level of
knowledge and describe the procedure of delivery in a more technical fashion, practices still followed the midwife's opinion and the customs and atti-

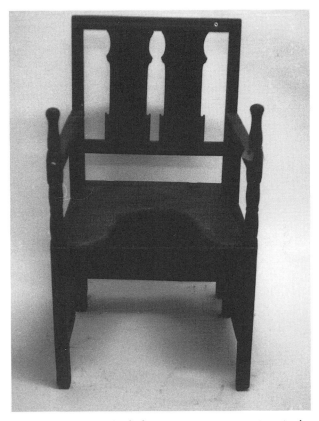

Figure 1.15. Folding birth chair, German, c. 1750–1850, in the collection of The National Museum of Science and Industry, London. Constructed of wood with iron hinges and brackets. The seat folds up onto the interior of the back and the sides fold inward for transportation. Photograph by author.

tude of the local community and had regard for the mother's comfort.

In keeping with the prevailing philosophy, during the hundred years following the publication of texts like those of Rueff and Rösslin, the basics of birth-chair design remained fairly consistent, although not without some aesthetic changes and alterations. Builders straightened, elongated, and squared the birth chairs' backs and sides and made the chairs' arms higher and the seat more rectangular. Two small posts or knobs were more consistently added at the ends of the arms so the mother had a place to grip. In addition, starting in the early 1700s, the majority of these chairs folded for portability and began to exhibit slightly higher seats, although the woman could still reach the ground with her feet. There are a number of extant examples of this style of upright birth chair, although simpler models still continued to be built and used as well.

For example, a European birth chair (c. 1700–1750) has lathe-turned legs, fixed hand-holds at the ends of the open arms, and a decorative crown-like design (Figure 1.14). The chair has a fixed, open back and a moveable seat secured in place by metal hooks attached to the underside that was secured in brackets attached to the interior side of the chair. This chair seat is seventeen inches from the ground. The chair folded for transportation. Likewise, a German birth chair (c. 1750) has a similar seat and folding design (Figure 1.15). The seat height is indicative of the growing trend toward higher seats, measuring twenty inches from the ground.

The Rise of the Profession and Changing Designs

In the later years of the eighteenth century, birth-chair design began to change. Thus, we may conclude that practices and, therefore, the overriding philosophy of birth began to change as well. Three significant developments provided the necessary influence and subsequently radically altered the natural philosophy of birth and the experience-centered, simple practice of delivery. The first and foremost was the development of the scientific study of obstetrics at universities. This began in Germany with the establishment of midwifery programs at Straßburg in 1728 and Göttingen in 1751. Institutions for teaching obstetrics quickly followed at universities in Berlin (1751); Vienna (1752); Braunschweig (1774); Detmol, Bruchsal, Dresden (1775); and Würzburg (1779). As educational opportunities arose, the writing of medical and obstetrical texts and treatises increased and new techniques were created and advocated.[37] These included the development of specialized tools for birth and the advent of the use of obstetrical drugs such as ergot and forms of anesthesia.

Second, although doctors were writing midwifery manuals and getting limited exposure to deliveries in hospitals for the indigent, when a doctor or a male-midwife was called to private deliveries, it was still only in emergency situations. If the mother had died, these practitioners typically performed a cesarean on the dead woman, or, in the case of impaction, they dissected the infant and removed it piecemeal from the birth canal.[38] However,

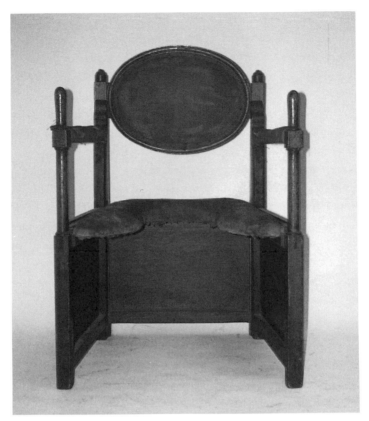

Figure 1.16. Collapsible birth chair, French, c. 1700–1830, in the collection of The National Museum of Science and Industry, London. This chair is constructed of walnut with iron hinges and pins and green and red velvet upholstery. The chair is 37.75 inches high, 25.25 inches wide, and 21.5 inches deep. The seat is 17 inches above the ground. For transportation, the sides detach and the seat hinges upward onto the back, which reduces the chair into three separate pieces. The chair is assembled when the back and sides are connected via latches and wing nuts and the seat is secured to the sides with hook and eye attachments. Photograph by author.

the advent of obstetrical forceps led to the more general employment of male-midwives in normal, non-life-threatening deliveries, thus improving their popularity by providing an alternative to the mutilation of the infant in the case of a difficult or impossible delivery. As Hugh Chamberlain wrote, use of the forceps dispelled the notion "that when a man comes, one or both must necessarily die."[39] Despite improvements in outcomes, doctors understandably gained a perspective of labor and delivery as a difficult and dangerous event. This attitude was a significant development because academic interest in delivery thus largely focused on the difficulties of labor and the birth of "monsters," infants with acute genetic deformities.[40] The texts of physicians became less directed to practicing midwives and contained more discussions of the fascinating aspects of labor and delivery directed toward their fellow physicians. The limited exposure of doctors to normal labor and the popularity of texts that dealt almost exclusively with abnormalities, such as poor presentation, impacting, narrow pelvises, and the birth of "monsters," cultivated an increasingly threatening picture of birth. This quickly led to a perception among doctors, and eventually among the population they tended, that birth was anything but normal. For instance, Hendrik van Deventer's *The Art of Midwifery Improv'd* (1728) devoted ten of its fifty chapters to "Difficult Birth" and eleven to various forms of poor presentation and other difficulties, along with an appendix entitled "Of the Birth of Monsters and Such Sort of Infants."[41]

The third development that altered the practice of delivery was that furniture design and innovation made possible many new designs of birth chairs. For example, a French birth chair (c. 1750) has a seat height seventeen inches above the ground, the classic seat opening, hand-holds, and an open back, but it also disassembles completely for transportation. The back, secured to the sides via nuts, bolts, and latches, breaks away from the sides and the seat hinges upward (Figure 1.16). Such innovations laid the groundwork and suggested the possibility of more radically altering birth-chair design.

By the early eighteenth century, more physicians were writing midwifery texts, attending in the case of difficult delivery, and even founding hospitals for the delivery of indigent women. The growing power and influence of the physician guilds and colleges increasingly became a real threat to the livelihood and status of midwives, as they competed for clientele and became less crucial to the care of the community. Through guild membership and the concomitant persecution of nonmembers who attempted to practice medicine, physicians and surgeons controlled and regulated the medical profession as they saw fit. Midwifery had come to the attention of medical specialists; doctors became interested in obstetrics and often the practice of midwifery.

As midwives lost their status, the traditional philosophy of birth began to subside as well. It was not only the midwife who was losing ground as an important and responsible member of the community. With the dismissal of midwives, women began to lose an important economic profession and their most accessible occupation.[42] The general status of women and their active role in childbearing deteriorated hand-in-hand with that of the midwife.

Although medical interest and the resulting redefinition of birth were certainly stimulated by doctors' increased exposure to birth, the fundamental motivation for this interest in birth was, at base, the development of a profession of medicine and the growth of the middle class, especially the discovery of middle-class women as a lucrative market for physicians. Such increased involvement of physicians in birth and the growing social acceptability of their involvement resulted in a rise in the prestige attached to the practitioners of official medicine, which in turn allowed the medical profession to increase its authority. Increasingly, as doctors gained control of midwifery and interpreted birth as a medical crisis that civilized women were unable to deal with appropriately, the systematic reinterpretation of the role of women and the medicalization of birth was accepted by the population that doctors sought to tend. This radical alteration of the social and cultural definition of birth, in turn, began to change the practice of birth.

Prior to the medicalization of pregnancy and delivery, folk religion and folk medicine had been the main forces in the philosophy of birth. Such changes in the overall cultural construction of the birth event came to characterize the late eighteenth and nineteenth centuries in both western Europe and in North America. As we will see in the next chapter, these attitudes were increasingly borne out in practice with the rise in invasive practices ranging from doctor attendance at birth to blood letting, anesthesia, forceps delivery, recumbent postures, and the eventual move to hospitals for birth. Birth became a private, medical event that required care and cure, which society began to believe a midwife was incapable of providing.

This process is vividly illustrated by the rapid and radical changes in birth-chair design. Birth chairs became more elaborate and technical; they were products not of the community, but of the practitioners of obstetrics. Birth chairs reflected movements in attitude, not functional responses to the event itself. These designs offered endless innovations that were defended in medical texts and accompanied by condemnation of other and earlier designs. By the early nineteenth century, works of physicians often lacked even specific discussion of birth chairs, but were instead devoted mainly to the abnormalities of birth.

Together, the interest in the medical aspects of pregnancy and delivery, the growing profession of medicine, the idealization and invalidization of women, and the ridiculing of the skills of midwives heightened the perception among the university-educated physicians, and eventually society, that birth was a dangerous and pathological event—a perception that systematically led to a practice of birth that was anything but natural.

Notes

1. This mode of delivery is also described in Margaret Atwood's *The Handmaiden's Tale*. In the novel the infertile wives of the elite have children through their handmaidens by having them deliver in this sitting posture.

2. Kilmer (1987: 211–213). Women also kneeled over these stones. This elucidates the narrative tradition in Cornwall of the presence of the handprints of St. David's mother on two stones near a well. According to the legend, she braced herself in this manner against these stones while giving birth to the saint. See Doble 1960–1970.

3. Thorwald (1962: 119).

4. Literally "upon the two stones." This word has a number of meanings in its use in the Bible. In Jeremiah 18:3 it is used as "potter's wheel" or "mill-stone." In its older form, it simply meant stone, as in Genesis 31:46 and Exodus 17:2. See Gesenius (1951: 7), Black and Rowley (1962: 210), and Elliger and Rudolph (1984).

5. Adamson (1985: 176–183). The style of birth stool depicted in this fresco is very similar to an Egyptian example located at the National Museum of Science and Industry in London. For another artistic example of a similar chair, see Croutier (1989: 111). These Greek and Roman items are in the collection of the National Archaeological Museum, Athens, Greece.

6. Hope (1893).

7. Englemann (1882), Jarcho (1934), Speert (1973).

8. Speert (1973: ch. 9).

9. Jonson (1914: 54).

10. Wilson (1990: 68–107). See also Crawford (1983: 49–85), Evelyn (1993: 9–26).

11. *Encyclopaedia Britannica; or a Dictionary of Arts and Sciences, Complied upon a New Plan in which The different Sciences and Arts as digested into distinct Treatises or Systems; and the various Technical terms, & 'c. are explained as they occur in the order of the Alphabet*, 1st ed. London, 1771.

12. As Jacques Guillemeau, the son-in-law of Paré (1540–1613) in *L'heureux Accouchement des femmes* (1609) (translated in English as *Childbirth, or the Happy Delivery of Women* [1612] stated, "It is very certain, that all women are not delivered after one fashion; for some are delivered in their bed, others sitting in a chaire, some standing

being supported and held by the shoulders or else leaning upon the side of a bed, table or chaire; others kneeling being held up by the armes." Guillemeau (1612: 88).

13. Judy Litoff (1982: 4) stated that for the colonial American population, "birth was deemed natural in that it was usually regarded in a matter-of-fact manner."

14. Van Doren (1963: 15).

15. Wehrli (1927: 95).

16. For more information on taboos and pollution see Douglas (1984).

17. Williams (1804: 3–4).

18. Fielding (1961: XIV: 51).

19. For example, a woodcut from Marcin Siennik's *Herbarz* (1568), a midwifery text from Poland, presents a midwife with a number of female attendants delivering a women seated in a birth stool or chair.

20. Radcliffe (1967: 7).

21. Raynalde (1540: 141–143).

22. Raynalde (1540). For publication and scholarly information about the translations of Rösslin's work, see Sir D'Arcy Power (1927).

23. "Darum ihr allerliebsten Frauen nach dem als ich gebeten bin worden von eüch, etwas zy schreiben den schwangeren Frauen, bitt ich Eure Liebe, das in keinem Argen aufzunehmen, wo ich zu grob wär gewesen; denn solches hab ich nicht um und um vermelden können." Bayerland (1910: 14).

24. Culpepper (1671: i). A recent reprint of Culpepper's work is now available. See Thomas (1993).

25. Texts such as Frontanus, *The Woman's Doctour* (1652); Wolveridge, *Speculum Matricis or the Expert Midwives Handmaid* (1671); Sermon, *The Ladies Companion, or the English Midwife* (1671); Oliver, *A Present for Teeming Women* (1688); Chamberlain *Midwife's Practice of a Guide for Women* (1665); the court midwife of Brandenburg, Justine Siegenundin, *Die Chur-Brandenburgische Hoff-Wehe-Mutter* (1690); Horenburgin, *Wohlmeynender und Nötiger Unterricht der Hebammen etc* (1700); and Mesnard, *Le guides des Accouchers* (1753) made extensive use of Rösslin and Rueff, but also included limited original discussion.

26. "My patient delivered at 8 hour 5 minute Evening of a fine daughter. Her attendants Mrss. Cleark, Duttum, Sewall, & myself. We had an Elligant [sic] supper and I tarried all night." Ulrich (1980: 127; 1990: 163).

27. Janet Carding, The National Museum of Science and Industry, letter to author, 1 May 1990.

28. For example, according to local tradition German women in Jachau in northern Bavaria, a rural area, used birth chairs as well. Unlike their urban contemporaries, however, they delivered in the main hall of the house. They did this because the hall was usually the original or oldest part of the house and therefore presumably the location of the sacred hearth. This is Wurnig's (1948–50) own example, although it contradicts his point. See also Giron (1906–1907: 38), Shorter (1982: 56), Gélis (1991: 130).

29. For example, Villerme (1821: 254) states, "Among the curiosities which were to be seen [in the eighteenth century] in the cabinet of the Grand Duke of Florence

was one of these chairs, decorated with jewels from top to bottom. Vanitas vanitatum." Quoted in Gélis (1991: 289, n. 53).

30. Judith Lewis (1986: 153–192) cites a number of letters and diary references to birth chairs and chair beds and arrangements between family and friends about borrowing these items to have on hand in preparation for delivery.

31. Bourgeois (1875: 108–109). See also Goodell (1876: 21).

32. Quoted in Robb (1893: 75–81).

33. In the Middle Ages midwives were required by law to baptize children, often in utero, in the incident of a difficult or fatal delivery. Thus, the church was interested in their standing as Christians more than in their skills in delivery. In addition, part of a midwives' duties, as dictated by church authorities, required their determining the identity of an illegitimate child's father. See Bancroft-Livingstone (1956: 263), Ulrich (1990: 147–149).

34. Furthering this association were the Dominicans Heinrich Kramer and Jakob Sprenger, who wrote in their 1484 *Malleus Maleficarum* ("Hammer of Witches"), "No one does more harm to the Catholic Church than midwives." Quoted in Donegan (1978: 11). In fact, the church-instigated *Malleus Maleficarum* went so far as to state, "If a woman dare to cure without having studied she is a witch and must die." Quoted in Ehrenreich (1973: 19). Historians estimate the total number executed during the European witchcraft craze (from the 1300s to the 1600s) to have been in the millions. Ehrenreich (1973: 7–8).

35. Various Christian doctrines loosely supported the interpretation of illness or death as the will of God or the result of sin and association with the devil. In fact, Rueff (1554: 10) believed that "monsters," children with deformities, were begotten by devils. By association, midwives were increasingly considered suspicious and vulnerable to charges of witchcraft with the failure to deliver a perfect child. The case against Mary Dyer and Anne Hutchinson in the Massachusetts Bay Colony is an example of this. See Tarter (1993: 22–26). Suspicion was particularly attached to their access to objects long considered "magical": the placenta, the umbilical cord, and the caul. For example, in 1555 Würzburg regulations for midwives forbid them to take away the placenta and required that they throw it in running water. As late as 1711 Brandenburg regulations forbid midwives to give away or sell any remains of birth like the membranes, caul, or umbilical cord. See Forbes (1966: 118).

36. Smellie (1779: I:203; II:168).

37. Radcliffe (1967: 32).

38. Bancroft-Livingstone (1956: 263). The term "accouches," by and large, was used in reference to male-midwives and appeared in the titles and texts of works beginning in the late eighteenth century. The *Oxford English Dictionary*, however, cites the first literary use of "Accoucheur," the French and, hence, polite term for obstetrician, as Lawrence Sterne's 1759 novel, *Tristram Shandy.* "—yet nothing will serve you but to carry off the man-midwife. —Accoucheur, —if you please, quoth Dr. Slop. — With all my heart, replied my father, I don't care what they call you, —but I wish the whole science of fortification, with all its inventors, at the devil; —it has been the

death of thousands." Literary commentary credits Dr. John Burton of York (1710–1771) as the victim of Sterne's satire. See Sterne (1940: 2:12, 113).

39. Forceps were invented in France in 1588 by Peter Chamberlain (1560–1631). Such forceps were shaped like two large spoons and were inserted into the birth canal once at a time around the baby's head and then screwed together. The infant was then pulled out. They were carried from one job to another in a large, locked, and highly ornate wooden box. When the Chamberlains arrived, the patient was blindfolded and the room darkened and only members of the Chamberlain family were allowed to enter the room. Bells and noises were made to muffle the noise of the forceps. Due to this secrecy, forceps were almost unknown until 1699, when the design was sold to a Dutch college. For more information on the development of obstetrical forceps, see Wilson (1995: 65–78).

40. While in the late Middle Ages and the Renaissance the association of a midwife with a child with acute deformities might bring about an accusation of witchcraft, the involvement of a doctor with such topics in this later period was a sign of medical expertise. Whereas a midwife was required to baptize an infant, doctors were called in to dissect and dismember. This alone indicates a significant difference in the perception of the birth act. What remained important, regardless of church- or guild-driven agenda, was that until the twentieth century, the life of the mother over that of the infant remained undisputed.

41. Deventer (1728: 320).

42. Carol Karlsen (1987) discusses the economic motivations for witchcraft accusations during the Salem witchcraft trials.

Curse or Cure?
The Rise of Professional Medicine, the Redefinition of Birth, and the Move from Chair to Bed for Delivery

By the turn of the nineteenth century, the general practice of delivery was strikingly different from what it had been a hundred years earlier. Increasingly, birth was something practiced rather than a natural event that occurred. This change reflected dramatic alterations in the overriding philosophy of birth, and this shift continued throughout the nineteenth century, with the naturalistic approach of the seventeenth century giving way completely to this medical philosophy.

While proof of this change in the cultural construction of birth is clearly evident in the shifting and altering practices of delivery, particularly as seen in birth-chair design, it is also apparent in changes in the field of professional medicine, the attitude toward women, and in the language regarding pregnancy and birth. A writer in *Gentleman's Magazine* in 1791 commented on this: "All our mothers and grandmothers, used in due course of time to become *with child* or as Shakespeare has it, *roundwombed* . . . but it is very well known that no female, above the degree of chambermaid or laundress, has been with child these ten years past . . . nor is she ever *brought to bed*, or *delivered*, but merely at the end of nine months, has an accouchement antecedent to which she informs her friends that at a certain time she will be *confined*" (emphasis in original).[1] By the mid-1800s, the use of such terms as "teeming" and "breeding" to describe pregnancy were replaced in contemporary diaries, literature, and other texts with terms such as "sick," "confined," and "ill."[2] In the titles of obstetrical texts, pregnancy and birth were increasingly referred to as the "diseases of women."[3] The texts written for women became little more than "advice" booklets for matrons, not midwives. These books instructed women as to the proper behaviors during pregnancy examinations and birth and provided general guidance for the selection and use of doctors.[4]

Although changes in terminology, practices, and birth-chair designs indicate a redefinition of the very idea of birth and a shift in the way it was understood to be best managed and practiced, the reasons for this philosophical shift are less apparent. Some historians argue that the changes in the practices of birth were the result of the growing fashion and acceptability of doctor attendance, the increasingly widespread use of obstetrical forceps, and the growing availability and dissemination of knowledge at educational institutions. Such histories, however, only categorize changes in actual practice and fail to associate such changes with larger ideological shifts occurring within society. Such histories convey the impression that changes in the practices of birth were the result of the growing acceptance of doctors and increased advocacy of their newer and better practices alone, without providing an adequate explanation for why and how this happened and detailing the other issues that brought about their attendance. These histories fail to take into consideration the general attitude of the populace toward women and midwives, altering societal (male) ideas about femininity and womanhood, the role of the raising middle class, the industrialization of Europe and the emphasis on the concepts of "progress," the changing professional needs of medicine, and the associated prestige and financial rewards of the medical profession.[5] In regard to changes in the actual practice of delivery, a purely technical history fails to consider how the above forces affected attitudes about the process and how these attitudes were then played out in practice.

That the practice of birth changed is obvious. By noting the way that these practices altered, it becomes evident that the philosophical shift systematically drove these changes. Specifically, the influence of attitudes affecting practice—form affecting function—is illustrated by changes in the design of birth chairs spanning this time frame. Each change in design reflected shifts in the social definition of birth and the role of women and their ability to bear children, and each design alteration resulted from some newly perceived medical need or understanding about the process. Each innovation reflected movement in ideology.

Thus, the changes in the practice of birth in the nineteenth century were actually the result of shifts in the societal attitude toward women,

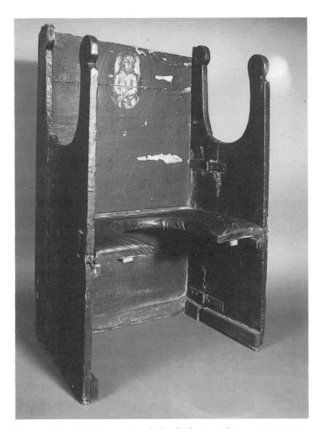

Figure 2.1. Folding panel-style birth chair, Italian, c. 1701, in the collection of The National Museum of Science and Industry, London. This chair is made of pine, painted green, with an icon of Jesus on the middle of the interior back and a seat covered in leather. The chair has been painted over on many occasions. The chair is thirty-seven inches high, twenty-three inches wide, and fifteen inches deep. The seat is fourteen inches above the ground. This piece was in the possession of a family of Sicilian midwives for three generations, until the late 1800s, and is estimated to have been used in 2,000 deliveries. After receiving a blessing by a local priest, the chair was believed to alleviate the labor pains of those who used it and became known as "The Miraculous Chair of Palermo." Photograph courtesy of The National Museum of Science and Industry.

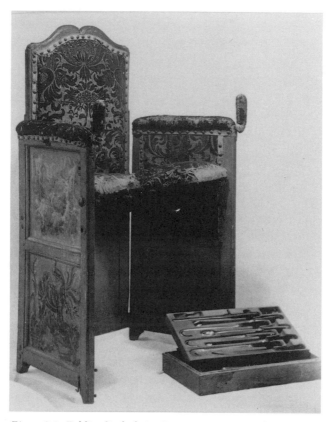

*Figure 2.2. Folding birth chair, German, c. 1800s, in the collection
of the Germanisches Nationalmuseum, Nürnberg. Upholstered in red
velvet brocade on the interior back, seat, arms, and sides. The external panels of the sides are painted with floral designs, principally the
pomegranate, which is considered a symbol of fertility. The chair is
42 inches high and 21.25 inches wide. There are three seat heights:
25 inches, 21 inches, and 18 inches. The moveable seat is secured in
place by two pins that fit through holes on the exterior of the sides
and into the side of the seat. For transportation the seat folds up and
the sides fold in. Unlike many chairs of the period, this chair, with
its richer finishing, was most likely the possession of a member of the
upper class. Photograph courtesy of the Germanisches Nationalmuseum,
Nürnberg.*

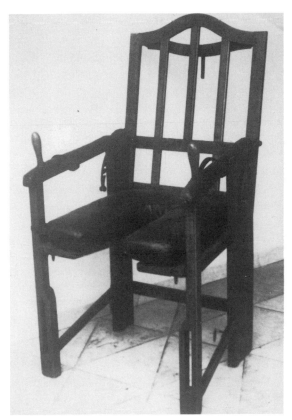

*Figure 2.3. Folding birth chair, German, c. 1800–1850,
in the collection of the Deutsches Medizinhistorisches
Museum, Ingolstadt. The chair has leather upholstery and a
removable leather pillow seat. It is 44 inches high, 24.75
inches wide, and 22.5 inches deep. The seat is 17 inches
above the ground. The back is attached to the sides via ratchets that can be lowered into a number of different angles from
the seat. A missing attachment, indicated by a wedge, would
have been placed under the lowered back for extra support. On
the lower front legs there are two braces that would have supported footrests, which are also missing. Hand-holds are fixed
on the ends of the arms. Leather straps attached to the arms
would bind a woman's arms in place, most likely during surgical delivery. Photograph courtesy of the Deutsches
Medizinhistorisches Museum.*

including notions of femininity, fragility, and competence; changing issues and needs of the profession of obstetrics, including prestige, financial reward, and authority; changing fads, fashions, and activities that affected the actual birth process; developments in medicine; and finally, how all these forces came together to form a new philosophy and cultural construction of birth.

The birth chair clearly mirrors this process, with the change in standard seat height being a prime example. Functionally, a lower seat was more practical because it allowed the mother to make effective use of contractions by bracing her feet against the ground. The ideas and attitudes of the new professional attendants, however, pressed for a higher seat, not because it was necessarily beneficial to the mother, but because it required less stooping and bending for the now more actively involved attendants. As Bernardion Ramazzini described in *De Morbis Artificum* (1713), midwives "attended always leaning forward and bent over, with hands stretched out, watching for the fetus to appear at the mouth of the womb they are so fatigued by all this effort and waiting . . . that when at last the infant is delivered they go home faint and exhausted, cursing their profession."[6] Whereas the midwife had seen her role as a community helper, the doctor was present as a paid professional.[7] He was, therefore, less inclined to inconvenience himself for a delivery. Whereas midwives simply went away clutching their backs and cursing their profession, doctors changed the height of the seat of birth chairs.

This is tangibly illustrated in birth-chair design changes over the years. From 1701, we have an example that is a simple panel chair with a low seat, which was reputed to assist and alleviate the pain of all who used it (Figure 2.1). From 1800, we have a German chair that offered three seat heights: twenty-five inches, twenty-one inches, and eighteen inches above the ground (Figure 2.2). By 1850, however, we find an elaborate German birth chair with footrests, a seat insert to close the classic semicircular opening, a ratchet back that afforded a number of back heights and angles, and, perhaps most telling, leather arm straps to secure the woman in place during delivery (Figure 2.3).

These changes in birth-chair design followed changes in philosophy and practice. Such design changes can be categorized as follows. First, the seat was significantly heightened. In 1513 Rösslin recommended a seat height of ten inches, and birth chairs dating from the 1700s typically had seats thirteen to seventeen inches above the ground. However, the birth chairs that came to characterize and set the standard in the 1800s had much higher seats. Second, to compensate for the higher seat, footrests were then added, which made bracing during contractions more difficult. Innovations in medical technology and practice, such as extensive use of forceps and other delivery tools and later forms of anesthesia, compromised the upright or semiupright posture of delivering women. Thus, new chairs featured backs with ratchets that could be lowered to accommodate a horizontal posture for delivery. In conjunction, the characteristic semicircular opening was often modified to include a piece that fitted over it to create something that was simultaneously a birth chair and a device with a closed seat that made it possible for obstetrical procedures to be performed. Hand-holds came to be considered less important than arm restraints and, often, leg restraints. Elements borrowed from contemporary "chairs of ease," or sick chairs, were added for effect, to the point that these chairs all but functioned as beds. Soon, table-like items replaced the chairs proper. Although these often maintained the opening, they wholly compromised the upright posture. By the turn of the twentieth century, birth chairs were reduced to delivery tables with stirrups, steel shoulder clamps, ankle and wrist restraints, and sterile field guards that separated the mother from the birth of her child.

As noted in chapter one, historically the experience of physicians had been primarily limited to only difficult or terminal births, which caused professional medicine to systematically understand and define pregnancy and birth as unnatural. As access increased through early indigent lying-in hospitals associated with centers of learning and city-funded hospitals, the number of professional obstetricians increased as well. As membership in professional guilds and organizations grew, doctors were driven by economic necessity to broaden their clientele. They accomplished this by increasingly defining birth as a dangerous, pathological crisis and thus undermining the credibility and compromising society's belief in the skill of midwives. Doctors increasingly portrayed birth as an event that warranted, in fact, demanded, their professional services and fed on the growing conception within society of the fragility of women. Physicians asserted the superiority of their profession and practice by creating specific medical terminology for the event, by introducing a liberal use of elaborate interventions and "necessary" tools, and by maintaining a monopoly over these.

Doctors and the Care of Women

By defining the process of childbearing as a disease state—a time of danger and possible death—and by contributing significantly to the perception that birth was an event with which women could not effectively cope, physicians taught society to view childbearing women and their "condition" as a sickness deserving medical attention and physician interest as a sign of their respect and concern for women. For example, in 1847 W. Tyler Smith stated, "The excellence of obstetric medicine is one of the most emphatic expressions of that high regard and estimation in which women are always held by civilized races. The state of the obstetric art in any country may be taken as a measure of the respect and value of its people for the female sex."[8]

However, contrary to physicians' assertions, the nature of their interest was twofold. First, midwifery had played an increasingly important role in the creation of a professional basis for medical practice. Second, professional obstetrical practice was key to developing a market large enough to support the growing number of doctors. According to William Smellie, when the British army and navy surgeons were put on half-pay in 1748, many of them began to attend his lectures on midwifery to increase their possible incomes.[9] Whereas doctors had earlier been content to dictate theoretical practices and procedures, the economics of the medical profession made it necessary for them to become more actively involved in the actual practice of midwifery as an entry into family practice. Simply put, doctors found that babies had become a point of good business. Walter Channing, professor of obstetrics at Harvard, wrote in 1820, "Women seldom forget a practitioner who has conducted them tenderly and safely through parturition. . . . It is principally on this account that the practice of midwifery becomes desirable to physicians. It is this which insures to the permacny [sic] and security of all their other business."[10]

Increased financial interest in women's health made it necessary to foster the appearance of utmost necessity. This encouraged physicians to develop and substantiate a definition of pregnancy and birth as a disease state. Doctors used science to supply a specific etiology and catalogue of symptoms, innovated invasive practices, elaborated birth-chair designs, and liberally used technologically advanced tools. As Walter Channing stated in 1848, when a doctor was called into a delivery he "must do something. He cannot remain a spectator merely, where there are many witnesses, and where interest in what is going on is too deep to allow his inaction."[11] Further motivation for the physician's strenuous activity during delivery was provided by the tragic story of Sir Richard Croft, who attended Princess Charlotte of England. Croft stood by watching as the princess labored unproductively for fifty-two hours, gave birth to a dead child, and then herself died; he then went out and shot himself.[12] By placing themselves in the public mind as necessary agents in the process for effective and safe delivery, doctors increasingly controlled and managed the birth act. Society responded by creating rewards and sanctions for their professional attendance. Consequently, the prestige of the practice of medicine rose steadily.[13]

Like Channing and Smith, most doctors insisted that civilization and the "bad habits of modern women" made a natural labor only "hypothetical." However, in 1895 Dr. Mary Putnam Jacobi clearly stated a more realistic reason behind the medicalization of birth: "I think, finally, it is in the increased attention paid to women, and especially in their new function as lucrative patients, scarcely imagined a hundred years ago, that we find explanation for much of the ill health among women, freshly discovered today."[14]

The necessity felt by medical professionals to increase their clientele to "practice" their art also led to competition among their fellow (male) practitioners.[15] Many resorted to name-calling, ostracism, and drumming rivals out of the various colleges and guilds of physicians and surgeons.[16] Because doctors could pass judgment on those of inferior ability, this unpleasant behavior had the effect of persuading the popular mind that there were high standards of medical practice.

Further enhancing their claim to superior skill and utmost necessity was the publication of countless obstetrical or midwifery texts by physicians, each of which advocated a regimen of practice during delivery, approved techniques, and recommend and regulated designs for new birth chairs. The sketches and recommendations for newer chairs further bear out the distinct difference in the way that birth had come to be regarded and practiced. Adam Elias von Siebold (1804), A. Schmittson (1808), and Anton Schmidtmüller (1809) recommended birth chairs of their own design and praised their own techniques as the best way. Schmidtmüller's design is so precisely presented and so elaborately detailed that it clearly stemmed from a conception of birth as an event to be directed, unlike the earlier texts in which the midwife was told to deal with birth as she saw fit. With adjustable footrests, arm restraints, a back that could be lowered to various angles via a side ratchet, arms that moved in parallel with the back, moveable hand-

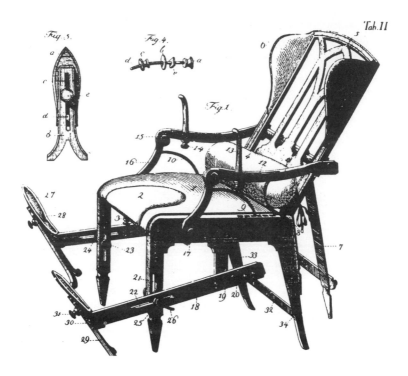

Figure 2.4. Sketch of proposed birth chair design from Johann Anton Schmidtmüller's Handbuch der medizinischen Geburtshulfe zur Grundlage bei akademischen Vorlesungen *(1809).*

holds, rabbit ears to frame the head, and a seat insert, this chair was strikingly different from the designs of earlier chairs (Figure 2.4). Schmidtmüller's design was not the product of a community, reflecting their varying attitudes about construction, design, and use and directed by the process of birth, but was rather the product of science, directed by the ideology of the attendant. As Ehrenreich and English note in *For Her Own Good: 150 Years of the Experts' Advice to Women,* "making something 'scientific' became synonymous with reform."[17] In 1811, Bernhard Christoph Faust went so far as to state, "Now my dear readers will agree that the Faust birthing bed is really the only one of its kind especially if its moral qualities are to be respected. As the Deventer birth chair once popular in Holland, such a talisman deserves its place in the dowries of all new brides."[18] Georg Wilhelm Stein went even further, praising his new chair and labeling all stools of midwives and others as "martyrs chairs and torture benches."[19]

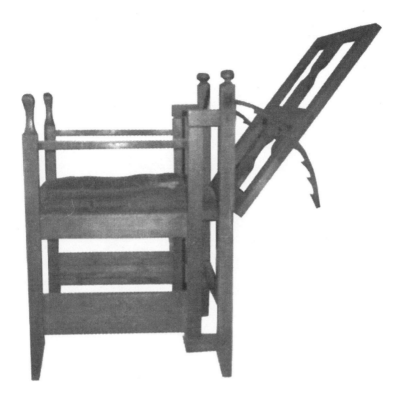

Figure 2.5. Folding birth chair, c. 1790–1850, in the collection of The National Museum of Science and Industry, London. This chair is made of wood with iron hinges and leather upholstery. The chair is 44.75 inches high, 25.5 wide, and 25.5 inches deep. The seat is 19 inches above the ground. The lower frame is grooved for footrest attachments, which are now missing. The seat folds upward against the back and the sides fold inward for transportation. The seat engages with sides via metal braces when folded down. The back is adjustable via ratchets, which are held in place by screws on the rear of the arms. Photograph by author.

The trend toward chairs advocated and designed by doctors quickly gained momentum, becoming so widespread that by the mid-1800s at least twenty-five different obstetric authorities in western Europe and North America had penned their own midwifery texts and were associated with birth chairs of their own design.[20] The similarity of extant chairs from this period indicate that the doctors commissioned local workshops to build their

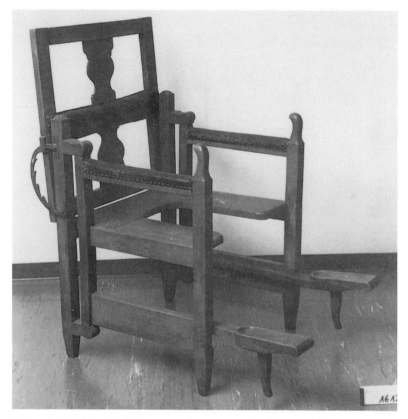

Figure 2.6. Folding birth chair, c. early 1800s, in the collection of the Medizinhistorisches Institut und Museum der Universität Zürich. This chair is made of wood with iron hinges, ratchet back, and leather upholstery on arms. The footrests are adjustable and remove for transportation. The chair is forty-four inches high, twenty-five inches wide, and twenty-six inches deep. The seat is twenty inches from the ground. Photograph courtesy of Dr. Christoph Mörgeli, Medizinhistorisches Institut und Museum der Universität Zürich.

designs and that these workshops then offered them for sale to the general public (Figures 2.5 and 2.6).[21]

Birth chairs became such an item of professional medicine that their earlier roots were all but forgotten. In fact, in 1802 Dr. Johann Gottfried Ebel stated, "For the last 20 years the doctors have been circulating instruction about the birth stool and now fewer women become sacrifices to sheer ignorance."[22] Not only had doctors taken over birth-chair design, construction, and use, they thought midwives were completely ignorant as

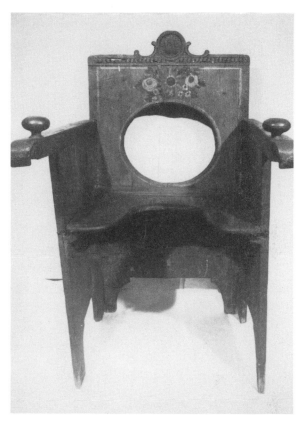

Figure 2.7. Folding birth chair, German, 1815, in the collection of the Thomas Jefferson University Archive, Philadelphia, Pennsylvania. This chair is in the panel style of earlier German chairs and has a circular opening in the back to allow access to the mother by midwives and assistants for massage and support. The seat is eighteen inches from the ground. It does not have any elaboration, except floral decorations on the external sides and an inscription "Dinzlau, 1815" on the external back. Photograph by author.

to their proper use. Although doctors were advocating their own special designs and were certain that midwives knew nothing of them (consider Dempsey's quotation at the beginning of chapter one), midwives were still active in this field. Midwives commissioned their own chairs (see Figures 2.7 and 2.8) and used them in practice, separate from the recommenda-

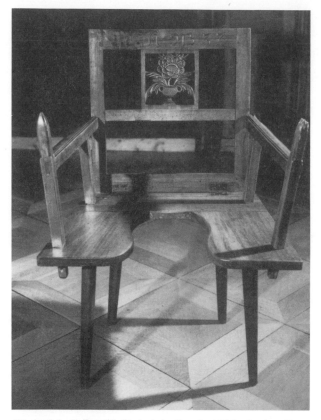

*Figure 2.8. Collapsible birth chair, French, 1830s, in the collec-
tion of the Musee Alsacien of the Musees de la Ville de Strasbourg,
France. The chair is 35 inches high, 25.5 wide, and 30.75 inches deep. The seat is 17.5 inches above the ground. This chair
breaks down into pieces for easy transportation. The seat is hinged
to the back, the sides come apart in two pieces, and the legs are all
detachable. The back is secured to the arms via hooks and eyes,
although it can be unhooked to bring the back into a completely
flat position if support is placed under the back. This piece is
thought to have been owned by a Jewish midwife practicing in the
area of Hurtisheim in the lower Rhine, Anne Willig, whose ini-
tials are carved on the chair back with the date "1837."
Photograph courtesy of Musees de la Ville de Strasbourg.*

tions and innovations of medical professionals and the advocated, newer
designs.

In response to the appearance of such authority and the presence of such seemingly advanced skill, society responded by accepting the medical perception and abandoning the older, natural philosophy of birth. Birth was no longer allowed to follow its own course, but was to be directed, controlled, and manipulated. This is evident in the practices of the nineteenth century that included the soon widespread use of obstetrical forceps and other delivery tools, the introduction of obstetrical drugs, bloodletting, the heavy use of anesthesia, the change in the role and gender of attendants, a more secluded atmosphere in the birth chamber, and new postures and styles of delivery. Such changes made the doctor physically more comfortable and enhanced his feeling and appearance of control, but simultaneously increased the actual burden on the mother and removed her control of the event.

Doctors' personal perceptions led to attitudes about what doctors would and would not do, how far they would be guided by a woman's preference and traditional approaches, and how much they would follow their own inclinations. This is clearly seen in a case history by Charles Meigs: "I was sent for to visit Mrs. C, whom I found lying on her right side. . . . I requested her to turn upon the left side, informing her that that position was the most convenient for me."[23] As with the alteration in seat heights, delivery practices were changed to ease the working conditions of the doctor, rather than those of the mother. Thus, the practice of birth was altered not by function, but by ideology.

These initial changes in the practice of delivery brought about by changing philosophy resulted in more innovations in the design and construction of birth chairs. As a consequence of the alteration in seat height, footrests had to be added to compensate (inadequately) for the loss of the woman's ability to brace herself against the ground. Although this alteration added to the difficulty of labor, extended seat heights and footrests came to be a standard item in the sketched designs and in birth chairs built from the early 1800s onward.

Such footrests would typically pass through slots on the inside of the front legs and would be secured by bolts higher up on the inside of the rear legs. In some cases, grooves on the interior stretchers of the legs held footrests in place. In many extant examples, although the footrests are now missing, they are indicated by the presence of these grooves or by bolt holes on both the front and rear legs. Footrests could be removed easily for transportation, and some were designed to be lengthened or shortened according to the patient's height. A German birth chair dating from c. 1800–1850, now owned by the Medizinhistorisches Institut und Museum

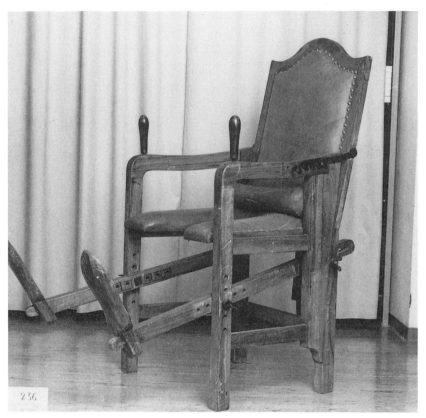

Figure 2.9. Folding birth chair, German, c. 1790–1850, in the collection of the Medizinhistorisches Institut und Museum der Universität Zürich. This chair is upholstered in leather with a small removable pillow, iron hinges, and ratchet back. The footrests are adjustable via bolts on the front and rear legs and remove for transportation. The chair is 46 inches high, 30 inches wide, and 36 inches deep. The seat is 19.5 inches from the ground. Photograph courtesy of Dr. Christoph Mörgeli, Medizinhistorisches Institut und Museum der Universität Zürich.

at the University of Zürich, has a seat height twenty inches above the ground and adjustable and removable footrests that offered six different length options (Figure 2.9). On the interior of the rear legs there are bolts that secure the top of the footrests to the rear of the chair, while the sliding grooves on the footrests allow for different lengths. On the front legs there are six bolt holes to likewise secure the footrests while allowing for height and length variations. The chair footrests (secured at both the front and the rear of the chair) attach via a long slot and butterfly bolts and can be adjusted in length. The foot patens are adjustable and offer three different sizes. While indicating signs of wear, this chair was finely constructed and upholstered in leather with a removable leather seat cushion. It was likely an item in use among the middle or upper classes. The similarity of this chair to the one now owned by the National Museum of Science and Industry in London is unmistakable. These chairs were most likely the work of the same workshop.

This medical inclusion and alteration of items and practices and the shifts in attitudes surrounding the birth process also encouraged the growing perception within society of women as fragile, inherently weak, unscientific, sentimental, and too uninformed to care for themselves alone—that women were, in actuality, exactly as they had been idealized.[24] Thus, women were perceived as being incapable of understanding and dealing with delivery. In 1825, William Potts Dewees of Philadelphia wrote, "[A woman] cannot fail to know less than her physician, therefore she is not entitled to be her own directress."[25] This is a striking and revealing example of the attitude that came to characterize the atmosphere in which women gave birth.

This perception and the changes in birth-chair design were not only caused by the increase in doctors, the development of the lucrative field of obstetrics, the progressive disintegration of society's confidence in women in the event of birth, and the reappraisal of women's health, in general, it was also fundamentally assisted by changes in the structure of communities due to industrialization and urbanization. The strong bonds of female community, which had been particularly noticeable through their participation in the delivery of a community member, were weakened by the movement of large segments of the population to cities and the increased isolation among urban women. In fact, pregnancy became an increasingly unacceptable topic of polite conversation.[26] People rarely spoke about birth; when they did, they used euphemisms and told "where babies come from" stories (e.g., the stork and cabbage patches). Even practitioners used such euphemisms when advertising their services.[27] Women spent most of their pregnancies in contrived seclusion and rarely spoke with other women on this topic. For example, S. Weir Mitchell of Philadelphia forbade his patients to speak about their condition with anyone but him. In 1888, Mitchell stated, "Wise women choose their doctors and trust them. The wisest ask the fewest questions."[28] However, the dialogue between practitioner and patient was quite limited. Women learned little about their condition, due to the instilled notion of

female modesty, society's acceptance of doctor's knowledge, and the perceived ignorance of women concerning the whole process of birth in contrast
to the advanced knowledge that doctors possessed.

Prior to the rise of obstetrical practice, use of the same practitioners (local
midwives) and the same techniques by both upper-class and lower-class women
had established what Adrian Wilson called a "collective culture of women."[29]
However, the social climate that separated "genteel" and lower-class women in
the nineteenth century also emphasized different approaches to labor and delivery, thus further limiting discourse and this "collective culture." For the upper
classes and those aspiring to that level, the blurring of the class line that similar practitioners would engender was portrayed as socially unacceptable.
Medical professionals cultivated this understanding, and their attendance and
techniques among the upper classes inevitably set a standard of care that filtered down the class structure as others sought to emulate their "betters."[30]

This movement was successful. Employing doctors for delivery, which
began to represent upper-class social behavior, became widespread and conventional among those classes able to afford it and even among those that
could not as a means of mimicking upper-class behavior.[31] As for concepts of
"female delicacy" and modesty that argued against attendance by any male,
doctors used class arguments to belittle and dismiss such sensitivities as
socially retrogressive thinking. As a country practitioner in Ontario stated
in 1875, "Are women of Canada more refined in their feelings or more sen-
sitive in their address than the Queen or the Princess of Wales and other
ladies of the Royal Family? They could have had the services of thoroughly
experienced midwives . . . yet they were all attended by professional men."[32]
However, the modesty of women as an argument against male practitioners
has not been borne out in history. As Wilson stated, "the concept of 'modesty' was a construct, not an embedded attitude; it was not of ancient lineage
but was produced in our period; and it emanated not from women but from
men."[33] As a created attitude, modesty was used by male practitioners to
explain why, if they were indeed the logical and natural agents for childbirth, they had been absent until only relatively recently.

The declining use of midwives, restricted communication among women,
and the growing physician monopoly not only of the market, but even of the
topic of birth, brought about a severe decrease in women's knowledge about
birth. Birth was removed mentally, physically, and conversationally from the
community. As Charles White stated in *A Treatise on the Management of*

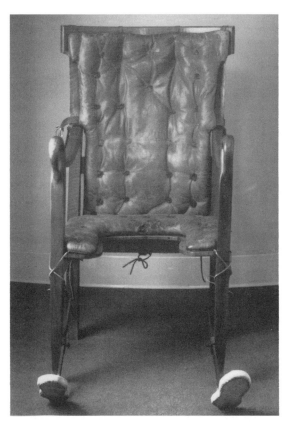

*Figure 2.10. Birth chair, German, c. 1750, in the collec-
tion of the Clendening History of Medicine Library at the
University of Kansas Medical Center, Kansas City.
Constructed of walnut with leather upholstery, this chair is
47.25 inches high, 19.5 inches wide, and 19.5 inches deep.
The seat is 17 inches above the ground. The back, seat, and
arms are fixed, and the chair does not fold for transportation. This chair was altered at a time after its original construction to included metal footrests with cloth-covered foot
patens. This piece was purchased for Dr. Logan Clendening
in Switzerland in 1935. Photograph courtesy of the
Clendening Library.*

Pregnant and Lying-In Women (1791), "As soon after the woman is delivered as it can conveniently be done, clean linen should be put around her, she should be left to the most perfectly quiet of body and mind, that she may, if possible, get some sleep. The child should be removed to another room, and no visitors, or other persons, except such as are absolutely necessary, should be allowed to enter the patient's chamber."[34] This is a stark contrast to the scene of family members and neighbors going in and out, greeting the woman and new child, and the feasting as described by midwife Martha Ballard in the late eighteenth century.

The effect of such societal, professional, and medical changes are visually apparent in birth chairs. The deepening pathological definition of birth led to an increasing tendency toward more interventionist practice of delivery. This was reflected in increasing elaboration in the design and construction of newer birth chairs and encouraged the modification of existing birth chairs to compensate for their seeming simplicity and, therefore, apparent inadequacy of design.[35] Thus, as they became an accepted or expected element of design, footrests were added to already existing birth chairs, regardless of the height of the seat or original design. An example of this form of adaption is a standard upright German birth chair (Figure 2.10). Purchased in Switzerland in 1935 as a collector's item and now owned by the Clendening History of Medicine Library of the University of Kansas, this chair is dated at c. 1750 and has a seat height of seventeen inches.[36] Sometime after the initial construction, metal footrests with cloth covered foot patens were bolted onto the chair legs at fixed locations.

Likewise, another late-eighteenth-century German birth chair (Figure 2.11) has a seat height of seventeen inches. However, it has had six holes drilled into the front legs and one bolt hole on each of the rear legs, presumably to secure footrests in place. This was almost definitely a later alteration because the holes are of rougher handiwork and there are no brace slots on either the front or rear legs to support and strengthen the footrest attachment and no slide slots on the inside stretchers, as in birth chairs originally designed with footrests. The addition of footrests to these chairs had no real function because the seats were close enough to the ground to allow for bracing. The addition of these pieces is significant in what they represent—a change in the perceived level of intervention and assistance believed to be required for a successful birth. Another example of the alteration of existing

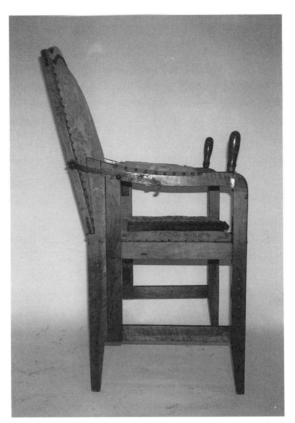

Figure 2.11. Folding birth chair, German, c. 1700–1850, in the collection of The National Museum of Science and Industry, London. This chair is constructed of varnished wood with iron hinges and braces and brass studs. It is upholstered in pink silk with a floral pattern and leather. The chair is 47.25 inches high, 23.5 inches wide, and 22 inches deep. The seat is 17 inches above the ground. The back, seat, and hand-holds are all moveable. The back is ratcheted and can be lowered to a number of different angles from the seat. The hand-holds have four settings along the arms to compensate for the different distances created by different back angles. This chair was later altered to accommodate footrest attachments, which are now missing. This is indicated by bolt holes of cruder workmanship on the front and rear legs. Photograph by author.

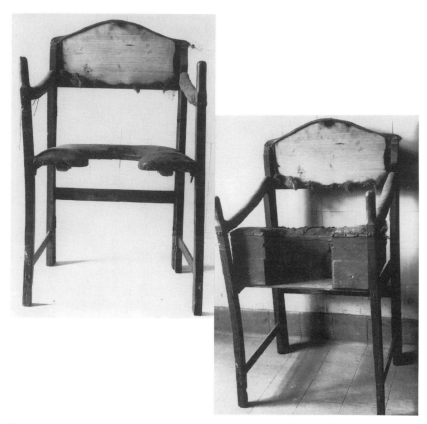

Figure 2.12. Folding birth chair, Austrian, c. 1750, in the collection of the Oberösterreiches Landesmuseum, Linz, Austria. This chair was last used in the Old Hospital of Linz. The back, arms, and the seat were once upholstered in leather. Although the back and sides are fixed, the seat is moveable and is secured in place by metal hooks on the underside of the seat, which fits into an eye attached to the interior side of the chair. A seat wedge built at a later date could be added to significantly heighten the seat to approximately twenty-eight inches above the ground. Photograph courtesy of Elfriede Priller, Oberösterreiches Landesmuseum.

birth chairs to bring them "up to speed" with their contemporaries for the sake of form, not function, is the later manufacture of a seat insertion piece for an eighteenth-century French birth chair (Figure 2.12). The chair has an original seat height of approximately seventeen inches from the ground. To enhance this height, a box seat, somewhat like a booster chair, was constructed to fit in place of the original seat (see Figure 2.12). This addition raised the seat height an additional six inches, presumably to make it easier for the attendant to observe the process of labor and adhere to the prevailing styles of higher seats. Such changes to seat height and the addition of footrests were seen as necessary alterations to make what was once considered an acceptable tool of birth useful again by meeting changing attitudes toward delivery and changing expectations of birth-chair design.

Idealization of Women and the Process of Delivery

Accompanying this increasing move toward devaluing women's usefulness and qualifications in delivery was the development of a parallel idealized social portrayal of women in general. As members of the growing middle class sought to emulate the wealthy classes in all ways, from doctor-attended delivery to showing that active economic participation of their wives and daughters was not necessary for their success, what had once been considered sinful was now a status symbol, idleness. Newspapers and magazines instructed every woman on how to elevate her status and that of her family by setting "proper" standards of behavior and taste. *Godey's Ladies Book,* as well as numerous others, preached piety, purity, and domesticity as the ultimate goal.[37] Idleness replaced usefulness, status replaced significance, and isolation replaced participation. This social movement had a stunning effect on the philosophy and practice of birth.

Associated with this "cult of true womanhood" were the arguments of many nineteenth-century doctors against female education and social involvement. They believed that not only did use of the brain detract from the normal development of those important organs of women, the uterus and ovaries, but it also significantly contributed to women's general poor health and the gradual appearance of mental problems. Medical and scientific researchers furthered the case by presenting alleged biological evidence of women's lower intelligence and of their inability to learn. For example, Paul Broca, a professor at the Faculty of Medicine in Paris, spent his life measuring the size of male and female heads and weighing their brains to find conclusive evidence that women were less intelligent. This was a common opinion. In 1879, Gustave Le Bon stated:

In the most intelligent races, as among the Parisians, there are a large number of women whose brains are closer in size to those of gorillas than the most developed male brains. This inferiority is so obvious that no one can contest it for a moment, only its degree is worth discussion. All psychologists who have studied the intelligence of women, as well as poets and novelists, recognize today that they represent the most inferior forms of human evolution and that they are closer to children and savages than to an adult, civilized man. They excel in fickleness, inconstancy, absence of thought and logic, and incapacity to reason. Without doubt there exist some distinguished women, very superior to the average man, but they are as exceptional as the birth of any monstrosity, as, for example of a gorilla with two heads, consequently, we may neglect them entirely.[38]

According to nineteenth-century doctors and scientists, education, exertion, and excitement caused irreparable damage to women's health. Thus, fragility and ill health became acceptable and common indications of refined sensibility and social status. Thus, if a woman did not experience illness as a result of such activities, she must not be truly female. So prevalent was this fashion of sickness that Catherine Beecher on her tour of 1871 decried "a terrible decay of female health all over the land." Her catalogue included: "Milwaukee, Wis. Mrs. A. frequent sick headaches. Mrs. B. very feeble. Mrs. S. well, except chills. Mrs. L. poor health constantly. Mrs. D. subject to frequent headaches. Mrs. B. very poor health . . . Mrs. H. pelvic disorders and a cough. Mrs. B. always sick. Do not know one perfectly healthy woman in the place."[39] Mary Livermore, a nineteenth-century woman's suffrage worker, went further than Beecher by denouncing "the unclean army of 'gynecologists' who seem desirous to convince women that they possess but one set of organs—and that these are always diseased."[40] Of course, illness was not only fashionable in relation to childbirth; often it became the only available means of control and power for women over their families and lives in a society that allowed women little visible means of power.[41]

The cultivation of upper-class women's ill health as a sign of status and civilized behavior further contributed to the growing conception, or misconception, that the whole process of childbearing was monumental, pathological, and well beyond a refined woman's capability. Society came to believe that birth was an area desperately in need of medical management and control. For example, in 1862 Edward Murphy stated, "In proportion as we remove women from a state of simplicity to luxury and refinement, we find that the powers of the system become impaired, and the process of parturition is rendered more painful. In a state of natural simplicity, women in all climates bear children easily, and recover speedily."[42] The social corollary to such thinking was that if a woman did not appear to suffer a difficult, possibly dangerous, labor and delivery, she was in action and demeanor like a savage.[43]

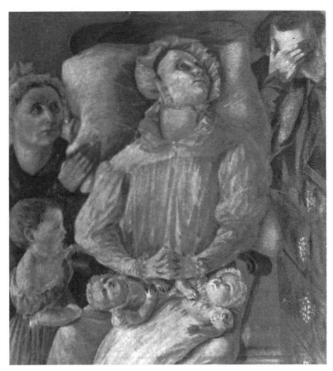

Figure 2.13. Death Scene, *c. 1841–1842, by Javis Hanks, in the collection of the Ohio Historical Society, Campus Martius Museum, Marietta. This work can be dated by the age of the surviving son (probably two or three years old in the painting). It is not a rendering of an actual event, but a recreation. The posing of the dead woman on what appears to be a birth chair is curious and telling. Reprinted by permission of the Ohio Historical Society.*

As doctors argued that delivery was a time of coming "down to death's door" and women complied with the societal requirements for indicating refinement, women relied more on doctors to protect them.[44] A classic example of this association with death in delivery is an example of a posthumous mourning portrait. Painted by Javis Hanks, *Death Scene* depicts Elizabeth Spencer Stone and her twins, who all died in the year 1840—one at five months, another at six, and Stone presumably at their birth. Note her posture and the chair she is sitting in—her legs spread apart, the posture of delivery on a birth chair (Figure 2.13).[45] Although the idealization of women and the fashionable quality of ill health was primarily an indication of upper-class sensibility, the standards of style were set and systematically filtered down in mentality, if not in action, to all classes.

However, the fashion of ill health among women and the professional understanding of birth as pathological were not the only elements involved in the redefinition of birth. During the nineteenth century, in some ways birth *had* become more difficult. While the idealization of women created an image of women as inherently unhealthy, life in the industrialized city, the often counter-productive changes in the practices of delivery like the use of higher seats and footrests, and the standards of what was considered fashionable dress in many ways made image reality. Years of use of women's undergarments and supports, such as corsets and straight lacing, seriously altered a woman's anatomy and made delivery difficult and often impossible due to a malformed torso and pelvic area, not to mention the damage done by continuing to wear them throughout a pregnancy (Figure 2.14).[46] In addition, the imagery of bound and tied women as represented by the corset is also very telling. In conjunction, the process of urbanization, which increased rapidly in the nineteenth century, cut off large portions of the population from fresh agricultural produce, sunlight, and physical exercise. This deprivation radically increased the rate of rickets, a nutritional disease that resulted in improper bone growth. Among women, this frequently meant malformed pelvises and difficulty in delivery.

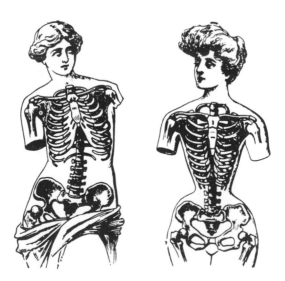

Figure 2.14. Nineteenth-century German sketch of the alterations in the skeletal shape and anatomy of women over years of corset use.

In addition, use of the newer designs of birth chairs also produced a domino effect of changes in the process of delivery. Chairs with high seats required footrests to compensate for the limited effective bracing during contractions. Despite these alterations, the higher chairs actually increased difficulty and complications in labor and were therefore related to the growing number of births now categorized as "difficult." This, in turn, increased what came to be considered necessary and appropriate control and management—use of obstetrical forceps. Thus, the standard upright birth chairs became less popular because use of forceps in the upright position was next to impossible. Therefore, chairs were designed to be both a birth chair and, with a moveable or detachable back that could be lowered into a horizontal position, a more bedlike apparatus. If the woman was laboring in a birth chair, it was more convenient to simply lower her into a horizontal position when forceps delivery was deemed necessary than to move her to a bed or onto a pallet on the ground.

Furthermore, the innovation of chairs with detachable or adjustable backs required a support or brace to prevent tipping. An early adaptation was the use of leather straps and hooks connecting the back to the arms of the chair. In such a design, the back could be adjusted by lengthening or shortening the leather straps that were attached to the back of the chair and then anchored by a hook to the front of the arm. When additional bedding was placed in strategic locations, these chairs could function as both a semirecumbent chair-bed for delivery and, most likely, a postpartum bed. This was clearly the original intention of the early lowering-back chairs because the hand-holds or grips could not be adjusted to accommodate the woman's changed position. If forceps were used, the woman would not be expected to want to labor during contractions and, therefore, hand-holds were thought to be unnecessary. Such innovations caught on quickly.

To better facilitate medical exams of laboring women and the use of delivery tools such as forceps and to make the lowering of chair backs more secure, later innovations provided iron ratchets on the backs of chairs to enable a variety of heights and angles and a more secure recumbent position. Ratchets were screwed to the back of the chair and the ratchet teeth would then be caught with a screw, pin, or bolt at the rear of the arms. By presenting the option of a variety of semiupright positions and styles, this adaption compromised the physiologically sound upright delivery posture, thereby adversely affecting the birth process. The hand-holds are moveable on such chairs, indicating that women did labor in these nonupright positions. An example of this style is a folding German birth chair (c. 1800–1850). Upholstered in leather with a removable leather pillow, the seat is seventeen inches above the ground at the lowest of its three seat options. The back is ratcheted and can be lowered into a number of different angles from the seat. An attachment, now missing, would have been placed under a lowered back for extra support.[47] On the lower front legs there are two braces and bolt holes for footrests (also missing) to be attached. The arms are fitted with hand-holds, and leather straps on the arms would have bound a woman's arms in place during surgical delivery. Because these additions made chairs larger, more complicated, and heavier, it became more difficult to fold them to be carried from delivery to delivery. Instead of folding, the newer chairs could be easily taken apart for transportation and then quickly reassembled at the proper location. This German chair breaks down into a number of separate pieces for transportation (see Figure 2.15), as did most chairs of the period. One design sketched by Friedreich Benjamin Osiander even provided a carrying handle for transportation, whereas another model fitted into a backpack for travel (Figure 2.16).[48]

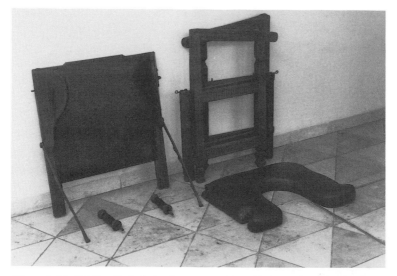

Figure 2.15. Folding birth chair, German, c. 1790–1850, in the collection of the Deutsches Medizinhistorisches Museum, Ingolstadt. Birth chairs broke down for transportation in this manner (see Figure 2.3 for the assembled version). Photograph courtesy of the Deutsches Medizinhistorisches Museum.

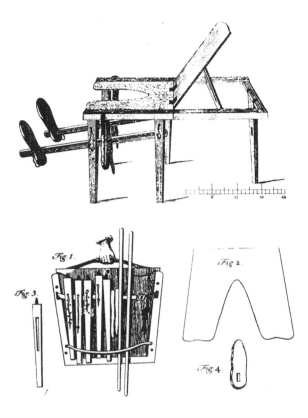

Figure 2.16. Sketch of a proposed design for a birth chair by Friedreich Benjamin Osiander from Osiander's Geburtsstelle *(1821).*

Although gaining in widespread acceptance at this time, the semirecumbent or fully horizontal postures for delivery were not inventions of the nineteenth century. These positions, outside of a birth stool or chair, had been an option in delivery since early times as a means to deal with a difficult delivery. What separated use of these postures in earlier periods was the rationale behind their use. Beginning in the early nineteenth century, obstetrical texts advocated horizontal or recumbent postures for *all* deliveries. The advocacy of these positions argues for a belief by medical professionals that all births were somewhat difficult. By the mid-1800s, such an understanding that births were routinely difficult was in place both in popular belief and in practice.

Furthering this argument, Laurel Ulrich compares birth statistics of Martha Ballard, a midwife practicing between 1785 and 1812 in Maine, with James Ferguson, a doctor practicing in the same area between 1824 and 1859. Whereas Ballard found only 5.6 percent of her deliveries "difficult," Ferguson found 20 percent of his deliveries "difficult." He described 102 as "tedious," 41 as "premature," 39 as "preter-natural," 33 as "complicated," and, after 1838, 31 as "instrumental."[49]

Later obstetrical histories rationalized this move toward the extensive and common use of a horizontal posture for birth as part of the effort to contain the spread of infection and disease. However, such postures became popular among physicians long before anyone understood the transfer of puerperal fever and other forms of infection and before the work of Lister and Pasteur. Statistics indicate that long after the recumbent posture in bed became popular, the incidence of puerperal fever continued to soar.[50] Rather, the use of recumbent delivery was based on physician's comfort, preference, and ideology and, eventually, on prevailing social styles. It is clear that the explanation of infection was created after the fact to explain and rationalize its earlier appearance. Also, medical histories of the day relayed stories of the first use of the recumbent position for delivery in bed. According to these narratives, the first use of a recumbent posture for a normal delivery (and in some versions, the historic first use of a male-midwife by choice and not necessity) was by Louis XIV's mistress, Louise de la Valliére, in the late seventeenth century. According to tradition, Louis insisted that she lie down so he could observe the birth (a socially inappropriate activity of the time) from his hiding place behind the curtains. Influential members of the French court then followed King Louis's lead and took to employing accoucheurs (man-midwives) when they wished to keep their illicit affairs a secret because part of a midwife's duties, as dictated by the authorities, required her determining the identity of an illegitimate child's father.[51]

In turn, what had been predicated on form became reality. Although far easier from the doctor's or practitioner's perspective, the horizontal position significantly increased the difficulty, length, and pain of labor and delivery.[52] Due to its contradictory influence on labor, the growing popularity of this position, in fact, encouraged the use of intervention and medical care and maintenance in the practice of birth. This, in turn, fostered the very understanding of birth advocated by the developing field of obstetrics. "Heroic" measures like extensive bloodletting and the administration of ergot and

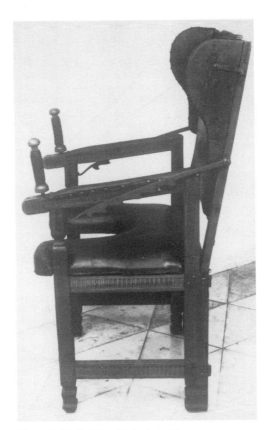

*Figure 2.17. Folding birth chair, German, c.
1790–1850, in the collection of the Deutsches
Medizinhistorisches Museum, Ingolstadt. This chair is
constructed of wood with iron hinges, back ratchets,
footrest attachments (missing), and leather upholstery.
The chair is 47.25 inches high, 25.25 inches wide,
and 18.74 inches deep. The seat is 19 inches above the
ground. The hand-holds are adjustable and rabbit ears
on the upper back can be opened outward or secured in
an upright position via hooks and eyes to frame and
support the woman's head. Photograph courtesy of the
Deutsches Medizinhistorisches Museum.*

opiates were regularly used in what midwives would have considered normal labors had then begun upright. These practices further encouraged the use of a recumbent position for delivery, use of forceps, anesthesia, and doctor attendance.

The results of such cyclical practices encouraged the understanding of birth as difficult and provided ample argument for the care and treatment of all deliveries by doctors as a medical crisis. The redefinition of birth and the resulting changes in practice made ideology reality. Significantly, the reclining posture, which is the posture of ill health, visually illustrated the definition of all births as sicknesses, as did the final "improvements" to birth chairs—the inclusion of elements of design such as moveable hand-holds and armrests, ratchet backs, and seat insertions. Such elements had been characteristic of "chairs of ease," or "sick chairs," since at least the early 1600s. For example, an invalid chair belonging to Philip II of Spain (1527–1598) had a hinged back, footrests, and a ratchet back, as well as casters on each leg so it could be wheeled around.[53] The appearance in the mid-1800s of aspects or elements of chairs used for the sick or elderly in birth-chair designs indicates a direct relationship with the growing conception of pregnancy as an illness that required maintenance, treatment, and cure.[54]

An early-nineteenth-century birth chair owned by the Deutsches Medizinhistorisches Museum is a perfect example (Figure 2.17). This folding German chair is so similar in dimension and style to an English "sleeping" or "sick chair" from the late seventeenth century (Figure 2.18) that it clearly illustrates the borrowing of elements of sick-chair design. This birth chair is upholstered in leather and has a seat nineteen inches above the ground, a ratchet back, separate footrest attachments, and pronounced and moveable hand-holds. Although the English "sick chair" also possesses a ratchet back and moveable footrests, the presence of a solid seat, a frame leg reinforcement across the front, and rods attached to the arms to support a reading desk make it clear that this was not a birth chair. Like the English chair, the German birth chair has detachable rabbit ears that could be opened outward or secured in upright position via hooks and eyes.

With time, the elements separating birth chairs from sick chairs, primarily symbolized by the classic semicircular seat opening, became even more blurred. For example, the "Ladies' Solace Chair" (Figure 2.19) described by Charles White lacked the characteristic seat and was so similar in style and design to contemporary sick or portable invalid chairs it is possible that

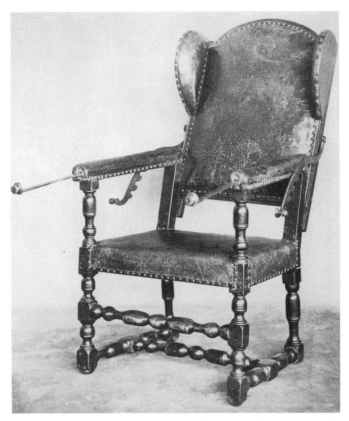

Figure 2.18. "Chair of Ease," or "Sick Chair," English, c. 1675, in the collection of the Victoria and Albert Museum, London. This chair has leather upholstery with rabbit ears, a rachet back, and solid panel footrest attachments. The rods inside the arms slide out to support a table for reading or writing. From Ralph Edwards, English Chairs *(1970). Reprinted by permission.*

many were used for both purposes, sickness and delivery.[55] With this blurring of the lines between birth chairs and the chairs used for the sick and elderly came the final blurring of lines between normal birth and birth as an illness.

Furthering this trend toward the popularity of horizontal delivery, the posture of ill health, and the understanding of all births as illness was the gradual transformation of birth chairs into "bed-chairs" or small tables, with delivery then being performed in the location of sickness, the bed. Additional pieces of seat were provided so that the semicircular opening

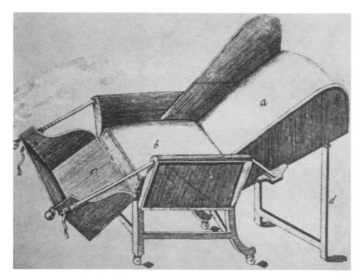

Figure 2.19. Sketch of the "Portable Ladies' Solace Chair," English, c.
1800, from Charles White's A Treatise on the Management of
Pregnant and Lying-In Women *(1791).*

could be closed over. Chairs were also designed with solid pieces of wood
that could be attached to the front of the seat or drawn out from under the
seat to provide a completely supported horizontal position when the back
was lowered. In such a way, designers of birth chairs sought to achieve the
best of both worlds—a birth chair that through design and additions would
serve as a bed. Designs sketched and scale models built were consistent with
these developments. Although these pieces were readily identifiable as birth
chairs, they were designed with an addition to close over the opening in the
seat and could be expanded to add length to the seat. Thus, they appeared
like and could function as a bed.[56]

The Degradation of Midwives and
Dismissal of the Tools of Their Trade

The alteration in the practice of delivery, particularly as evidenced by the
changing design and intent of birth chairs, was not the only element indicative of the growing influence of the pathological philosophy of birth and a
growing conception of the necessity of medicalized approach to delivery. In
concert with the redefinition of birth, the presentation of advanced skill, and

the heavy use of interventionist items and techniques, medical professionals resorted to the systematic repudiation of the remaining elements of the traditional philosophy of birth, midwives and the birth chair.

As rivals, midwives were portrayed in both scientific and popular literature as dirty, cruel, and incompetent. Charles Dickens's description of a midwife in *The Life and Adventures of Martin Chuzzlewit* was typical and reflected his cultural milieu: "The face of Mrs. Gamp—the nose in particular—was somewhat red and swollen, and it was difficult to enjoy her society without becoming conscious of a smell of spirits. Like most persons who have attained to great eminence in their profession, she took to hers very kindly, insomuch, that setting aside her natural predilections as a woman, she went to a lying-in or a laying-out with equal zest and relish."[57]

Not only did midwives represent competition for lucrative patient care, they were particularly troublesome because they typically delivered the children of poor or immigrant women, the very patients doctors wanted for use as clinical examples in obstetrical or lying-in hospitals.[58] Charles Zeigler complained in the *Journal of the American Medical Association,* "It is at present impossible to secure cases sufficient for the proper training in obstetrics, since seventy-five percent of the material otherwise available for clinical purposes is utilized providing a livelihood for midwives."[59]

The late nineteenth century was further characterized by vocal and continued debate about the role and effectiveness of midwives, their rightful or harmful place in delivery, and the systematic efforts of the profession of medicine to legislate, license, and consolidate physicians' hold over all avenues of medicine.[60] In her discussion of the decline of midwives in Quebec, C. Lesley Biggs describes the concerted movement of professional medicine against the practice of midwives that occurred at the same time as in continental Europe. She cited an 1845 editorial in *The British American Journal of Medicine and Physical Science* that fully captures the changing attitude toward midwives and their practice: "And when we consider the enormous errors which they [midwives] are continually perpetuating and the valuable lives which are frequently sacrificed to their ignorance, the more speedily some legislative interference is taken with respect to them, the better for the community at large."[61]

Thus, through active, technical involvement in delivery and the systematic repudiation of midwives, physicians argued for the necessity of their attendance, thereby altering any remaining notion in society that "if an uneducated woman of the lowest classes may practice obstetrics . . . it must require very little knowledge and skill—surely it cannot belong to the science and art of medicine."[62] The process of the exclusion of midwives from practice in North America mirrored the situation in western Europe, with midwives keeping some level of involvement only by moving their practice into hospitals under the tutelage of doctors and in strict adherence to the medical philosophy of birth. In North America midwives fared worse, with their wholesale exclusion as the prime objective of physicians.[63] Charges of illiteracy were equated with incompetence, use of traditional practices with ignorance, and the use of birth chairs with narrow-mindedness. As expected, a significant decline in the practice of midwifery by women was the response.[64]

In conjunction with the systematic degradation of midwives was a movement to repudiate all things associated with traditional midwifery and any practice of delivery termed "unscientific." For example, W. Tyler Smith was intent on eliminating the very word "midwife" from the language. In 1849 he stated, "We may confidently hope that hereafter the sign of the escape of midwifery from the midwife will be . . . that the term midwifery will be rejected on account of its derivation."[65] In fact, his favored term, "obstetrician," was the nineteenth-century derivation of the old Latin word for midwives, "obstetrix."[66]

The campaign against all elements of midwifery and nonmedicalized birth quickly moved beyond repudiation of midwives and the large-scale alteration, renovation, and elaboration of birth chairs to the rationalized dismissal of birth chairs altogether as antique tools of uninformed lay practitioners. Doctors discredited and maligned the advantages of birth chairs and focused instead on the convenience and "comfort" of delivering horizontally. The use of the birth chair faded in deference to the needs of the profession to symbolically separate from the past. As one obstetrical historian stated in 1937, the birth chair's "vogue died out and with the gradual elimination of the midwife, this relic of antiquity, too, has ceased to exist. Thus ended the dominance of midwives in the process of birth."[67]

Friedreich Benjamin Osiander and his son, Johann Friedreich, are representative of this shift toward a monitored and medicalized practice of horizontal birth in bed. The elder Osiander provided sketches of various styles and designs of birth chairs that he promoted. However, his son abandoned the birth chair of his father and others in favor of the use of forceps and delivery in a recumbent posture in bed.[68] While the early opponents of birth chairs condemned their use, stating that birth chairs would bring on a long and tedious labor and exhaust the mother, later critics claimed the opposite. Johann Friedreich Osiander, along with others, insisted that birth chairs produced too rapid and forceful a birth. They instead favored the lengthening of labor that resulted from a horizontal method of delivery.[69] According to some birth-chair opponents, those who believed in the effectiveness of birth chairs believed in fiction. As J. F. Schweighüser stated in 1817:

If a woman were to give birth alone without any assistance, she would not give birth sitting or standing. She would be led by nature to seek out or prepare a soft pallet and thereby secure protection of the perineum. Therefore, giving birth on a chair is against nature and to be wholly rejected. If when giving birth in this fashion the perineum does not tear, it is not to be attributed to the capabilities of the midwife, but rather to the course of nature. It is a completely false assumption that the woman giving birth on a chair can hold herself better and therefore, give birth more easily and more quickly. The only thing to be gained by using the birth chair is that the bed is not gotten dirty and for this reason there is great opposition to getting rid of the birth chair.[70]

Johann Friedreich Osiander went further in his ridicule and condemnation of birth chairs: "The birth chair is nothing other than a protection against the dirtying of the bed clothes and for this reason it is especially popular with stingy women and women of little means. The majority of women bearing children reject the birth chair because they cringe at the great tribulations of putting it together, lying upon it, and at the many other complications and unpleasantness involved with it."[71]

Earlier advocates of the birth chair lost their conviction in the face of denouncements by later obstetrical authorities of the "arbitrary" alterations in design, unsanitary situations, poor labor, and the even poorer working conditions. Even the elder Friedreich Benjamin Osiander had stated, "My objection to the use of birth chairs in private practice comes from the fact that I have often found the chair to be of faulty craftsmanship and to have been arbitrarily changed by midwives. I am, therefore, of the opinion that such an unhelpful machine, upon which the blood and sweat from the previous birth is still to be found, is not only counterproductive for delivery, but also is more trouble than it is worth to the one assisting the birth."[72] However, the fact that the majority of the alterations were initiated and directed by doctors and often caused difficulty in delivery was not discussed.

Later doctors argued that birth chairs were not only ineffective as a birth tool and were the items of the uninformed, but also that their use hindered the field of obstetrics from moving forward. In fact, in some areas authorities took steps to make use of birth chairs illegal, as in Malta in 1883.[73] As Lukas Boer (1751–1831), the head of midwifery at the University of Vienna, wrote, "the greatest service is the ban of the birth chair from birthing rooms and institutions."[74] Whether he regarded this dismissal of birth chairs as the saving grace of the medical professional or the safety of women is open to question.

By the late nineteenth century these former tools of birth were essentially all but beds and the understanding of birth that had driven such a change was a medical, pathological definition. This transition between birth chairs and the use of chair-beds and even regular beds for delivery and the associated change in the understanding and cultural construction of birth is clearly and distinctly captured in a "Gebärstuhlbett," a birth chair-bed that was constructed and used in Güntersloh in the area of Eifel, Germany, in the late nineteenth and early twentieth centuries.[75] Although still maintaining the characteristic opening to allow for passage of an infant during delivery, it sits like a table approximately three feet above the ground and the opening could be covered for a period of recovery or during surgical delivery (Figure 2.20). The legs are detachable for transportation from delivery to delivery. According to museum records, the last midwife who owned this device would travel to deliveries on her bicycle, bringing it along. (Judging from the weight of this table, she must have been a robust woman indeed!) Although this item was primarily used by a midwife, its design as a chair-bed reflected the closing gap between the practice of traditional midwifery and a confirmation of the newer attitudes and ideals of professional obstetrics. Although there were birth chairs of simpler design used by midwives in the early nineteenth century we cease to see this occur, thus indicating the eventual acceptance of these professional ideas.

Reflecting further this transition from birth chairs to bed delivery is a "birthing table" from England (c. 1890) from the design firm of Roginson and Sons (Figure 2.21). Dating later than the Güntersloh birth chair-bed, this table was a transportable delivery device, yet it lacked the defining element of a birth chair, the semicircular opening in the seat. The table measures six feet in length when expanded, and the back can be placed in seven different positions, including a completely horizontal position. The early chair-beds and "little bed" designs of von Siebold and Faust, which were followed by the Güntersloh table and this English example, clearly illustrate

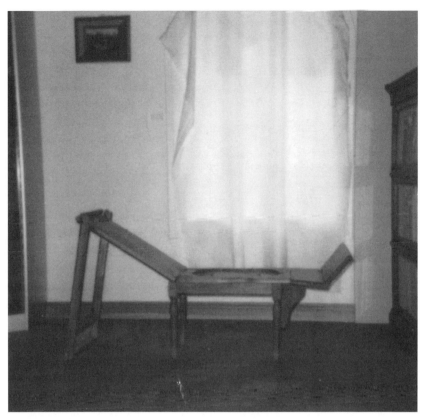

Figure 2.20. Birth chair-bed, German, c. late 1800s, in the collection of the Stadtmuseum Gütersloh, Gütersloh, Germany. This table is divided into three pieces that fold together for transportation. The legs are detachable. The chair-bed stands approximately three feet above the ground. As the back, one section can be situated into various angles, from upright to horizontal, from the seat. This chair was constructed and used by a midwife in the region of Eifel near Cologne and Aachen in the North Rhine–Westfalia region. Photograph courtesy of the Stadtmuseum Gütersloh.

the evolution of birth-chair design, the associated approaches to birth, and the prevailing philosophy behind such practices.[76]

Birth-Chair Designs and the Practice of Gynecology

Curiously, while doctors and medical professionals were strenuously arguing against the use of birth chairs in all deliveries, insisting on the dangerous, unhygienic, and primitive nature of the artifacts and those who used them,

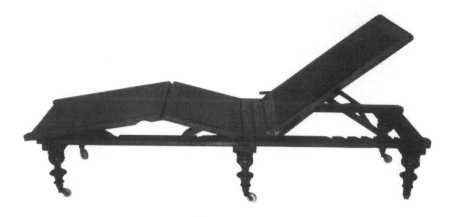

Figure 2.21. Birth or early delivery table, English, c. 1860–1880, in the collection of The National Museum of Science and Industry, London. The table is six feet long and is divided into three separately moveable sections. The back can be placed at six different angles or can be brought into a completely horizontal position. This piece was used until the late 1950s and was donated to the museum in 1983. Photograph by author.

the very design of birth chairs was being co-opted and utilized in the burgeoning field of obstetrics and gynecological care. Doctors that specifically dealt with women's "complaints" were cultivating a growing specialty, and the artifacts of their offices, the new "gynecological exam chairs," appeared very similar to birth chairs. They were so similar, in fact, that many were used for delivering infants, although not by doctors, but by midwives who came to possess such items. An example of this blurring of the lines between birth, delivery, and exams were the "Voltaire Chairs," which were constructed by Masion Dupont in Paris in the mid-nineteenth century. One such chair, owned by the Barcelona Museum of the History of Medicine, appears to be a simple drawing room chair with open arms upholstered in yellow velvet with foot casters and ornamentation. It is designed to convert into an examination chair, with a significantly heightened seat, foot braces, and a storage box under the original (the drawing room chair) seat, and it possesses a ratchet back. According to the museum director, this chair was designed and used for hysterometry—the practice of sounding the uterus—and other gynecological examinations, but was not used as a birth chair.[77] However,

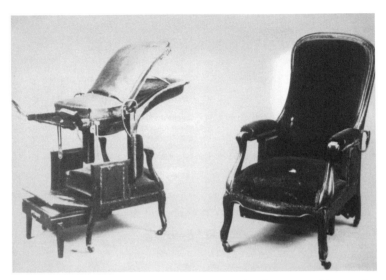

Figure 2.22. "Voltaire Chair," French, c. 1850. This chair was used by a midwife in Tours in the Loire Valley and by a local surgeon. It was designed to fold into itself, thus converting to a parlor chair when not in use (right). Reprinted by permission of Christie's South Kensington.

another "Voltaire Chair," which was most likely manufactured by the same company, was used for deliveries in Tours in the Loire Valley by the local midwife (Figure 2.22). This chair has green velvet upholstery and is believed to have been occasionally used by the local surgeon as well as by the midwife who owned it.[78] These items exemplify the blurring of lines between the uses of the artifacts of birth and gynecology as well as the important design roots of later obstetrical and gynecological exam chairs.

The Twilight Years

By the close of the nineteenth century, the balance of power and the philosophy of birth had completely shifted: Obstetrics had arrived as a legitimate branch of medicine, a field almost entirely dominated by men, and the process of birth was regarded as a pathological illness and was practiced as such. The peak of this shift in the philosophy of birth was the transition from an upright posture for delivery in a birth chair to a horizontal position, the posture of ill health, in bed or on a bedlike table device.

As we have seen, the impact of this medicalized philosophy of birth on the actual practice of delivery was so forceful that ideology drove the construction of birth artifacts, thereby tangibly affecting the practice of birth. Such a representative change supported the broadening definition of all births as "difficult," the creation of an ideal of women as inherently weak and unhealthy, and a pervasive understanding of birth as an event that required extensive, professional assistance to be successfully completed. The new approaches, practices, and artifacts of birth also clearly illustrate that women, who were once considered competent enough to manage the birth act, were systematically removed from it through the general idealization of femininity, growing pathological definitions of pregnancy and birth, seclusion during pregnancy, lack of education and communication with other women, and, finally, through the use of tools, drugs, and surgery. The birth act was achieved not with the mother, but for her.

Functionally, such changes were primarily a result of the growing popularity of the use of tools and narcotics in birth, which resulted in the growing use of horizontal or recumbent delivery. Ideologically, such changes were primarily the result of changing opinions about women and medical professionalism and these changes served the efforts of doctors to symbolically separate themselves from earlier midwifery practice. At root, these changes in birth chairs and in delivery practice illustrate that the driving forces were not changes in actual knowledge and improvements in the practice, but changes in the attitudes and beliefs of the principal birth practitioners and, subsequently, among the communities they tended.

Notes

1. Quinlin (1941: 67).
2. These terms are telling in their imagery of entrapped womanhood in the nineteenth century.
3. Such book titles include John Burns, *The Principles of Midwifery, Including the Diseases of Women and Children* (1810); A. Curtis, *Lectures on Midwifery and the Forms of Disease Peculiar to Women and Childrren* (1841); Fleetwood Churchill, *On the Diseases of Women Including the Diseases of Pregnancy and Childbed* (1852).
4. For example, see Buchanan (1815).
5. See Davis-Floyd (1992), Wilson (1995).
6. Charles White (1791: 29).

7. A midwives' prayer from the sixteenth century asks that she fulfill these expectations, being made, "wise-harted, skillfull, loving, gentle, tender, pitifull, willing, carefull, diligent, & faithfull, even for thy sake onelie, without respect of filthie lucre, to pleasure all women at all times in my calling, to the full discharge of my conscience and dutie, both before thee and the world." Bentley (1582: 135). Quoted in Charlotte Otten (1993: 20).

8. W. Tyler Smith (1847: 451).

9. Radcliffe (1967: 29).

10. Channing (1848: 223).

11. Channing (1848: 229).

12. Antony Smith (1968: 145). For more discussion of this case see Judith Lewis (1986: 85–121).

13. It was standard practice among doctors to charge twice their normal fee if a midwife had been called in to attend a delivery before they were called. Rosen (1946).

14. Cott (1977: 307).

15. See Vogel (1980).

16. See Averling (1882), Gevitz (1988: 1–28).

17. Ehrenreich and English (1978: 69).

18. "Meine schönen Leserinnen werden nun einsehen, daß das Faust'sche Geburtsbett wirklich das einzige seiner Art und vor allenwenn seiner moralischen Qualitäten hoch zu achten sei ein solcher Talisman verdient wie ehemals in Holland der Deventer'sche Geburtsstuhl künftighin einen Platz unter dem Brautschatze aller Neuver-mählten." Faust (1811: 45).

19. Quoted in Stucky (1965: 27).

20. For example, Hendrik van Deventer, *Observations Importantes sur le Manuel des Accouchements* (1701); Bernhard Christoph Faust, *Gedanken über Hebammen und Hebammen-anstalten auf dem Lande* (1784); Lorenz Heister, *Institution de Chirurgie* (1770); Jacques Mesnard, *Les guide des Accouches* (1753); Ambroise Paré, *Oeuvres* (1821); Georg Wilhelm Stein, *Kurze Beschreibung eines neuen Geburtsstuhls und Bettes* (1772); Christopher Völter, *Neueröffnete Hebammenschule* (1722).

21. The similarity of a chair from the mid-1800s owned by the National Museum of Science and Industry and another chair from the same period owned by the Medizinhistorische Institut und Museum der Universität Zürich argues for the work of the same manufacturer, as does the similarity between two period German chairs, one owned by the National Museum of Science and Industry and another in the collection of the Deutsches Medizinhistorisches Museum.

22. "Seit zwanzig Jahren werden Gebrauschsanleitungen für den Gebärstuhl von Ärzten verteilt und nun werden weniger Frauen Ofpen der reinen Unwissenheit." Ebel (1802: 291).

23. Meigs (1852: 174).

24. Baker-Benfield (1976). See also Cott (1977).

25. Hoffert (1989: 71).

26. See Smith-Rosenberg (1975: 1–29).

27. An example is a nineteenth-century French midwife's signboard, where a midwife is depicted bending over a cabbage patch where a number of smiling babies rest. Cuisenier (1977: Fig. 231). See also Bernstein (1976: 31–25).

28. Mitchell (1888: 48). Mitchell was the doctor who treated Charlotte Perkins Gilman to her "rest cure" and inspired her novel, *The Yellow Wallpaper*.

29. Wilson (1995: 38). See also Wilson (1995: 185–195).

30. Biggs (1990: 25).

31. Judith Lewis (1986).

32. Letter by "a country practitioner," *The Globe*, 11 September 1875. Quoted in Biggs (1990: 25).

33. Wilson (1995: 200).

34. Charles White (1791: 104).

35. Martin (1987: ch. 4).

36. E. P. Goldschmidt, E. P. Goldschmidt & Co. Ltd., London, letter to Dr. Logan Clendening, 30 September 1935 in the archives of the Clendening History of Medicine Library, The University of Kansas. Susan B. Case, Rare Books Librarian, Clendening History of Medicine Library, The University of Kansas, letter to author, 6 August 1992.

37. Welter (1966: 152).

38. Quoted in Gould (1980: 155).

39. Parker (1972: 165).

40. Cott (1977: 292).

41. See Wood (1973: 25–52).

42. Murphy (1862: 183).

43. Furthering this association was Englemann's *Primitive Birth* (1882). Englemann, convinced of the physiological benefits of upright labor and birth over the popular recumbent styles of his day, gathered together an extensive collection of illustrations, textural reference, and ethnographic accounts of various postures of birth throughout the world. His account did not alter the accepted posture. Instead it encouraged a connection between upright or squatting postures with primitiveness or "savages." See also Ashford (1988).

44. See Leavitt (1982: 113–136).

45. An oil painting, *The Visitation,* by the Danish artist Wilhelm Nicolai Marstrand dating from the mid-1800s depicts a similar chair. Here a healthy woman receives callers after her delivery. The chair on which she sits clearly has rabbit ears and ratchets and was most probably the style of chair that women of her day would have delivered upon. See Speert (1973: ch. 4).

46. For more information see Kunzle (1982).

47. Although now missing in some examples, many of these prop pieces are indicated by wedges and pins still present on the rear of the backs.

48. Stucky (1965: 24–25). A similar birth chair is located in the collection of the Medizin-Historischen Institute of the University of Zürich.

49. Ulrich (1990: 171).

50. Kosmark (1938: 8).

51. Bancroft-Livingstone (1956: 263).

52. See Cottrell (1986: 364–367).

53. Thornton (1978: Figs. 172, 173).

54. For more information on sick chairs or chairs of ease, see Bivins and Welshimer (1981), Thornton (1980: Figs. 72, 74, 201). Robert Trent of Winterthur Museum in Delaware has also done work on chairs of ease. For example, see Trent (1991).

55. See Drinker's "Ladies Solace Chair," in Drinker (1937: 171).

56. In 1791 John Christopher Stark introduced a design of lighter, curved arms and footrests with no moveable back. George Wilhelm Stein of Marburg (1731–1803) soon followed by sketching a chair that disassembled, had a moveable back, and a panel to close over the opening. Such as closure of the seat would quickly turn a birth chair into a postpartum or recovery bed.

57. Dickens (1915: 131).

58. Roberts (1981: 18–49). See also Vogel (1980).

59. Quoted in Ehrenreich and English (1978: 95).

60. Biggs (1990: 23).

61. An editorial appearing in *The British American Journal of Medicine and Physical Science* 1 (1845): 195. Quoted in Biggs (1990: 23).

62. De Lee (1916: 1126).

63. For further information about this phenomena in the United States, see Leavitt (1986); for Great Britain, see Donnison (1988), Towler and Bramall (1986), Wilson (1995); for Canada and North America, see Biggs (1990); for Spain, see Ortiz (1993); for Ireland, see Browne (1995), although this offers less criticism of the medicalization of birth. The movement is also reflected in Australia; see Willis (1994).

64. The Philadelphia city directory in 1815 listed twenty-one women as midwives and twenty-three men as practitioners of midwifery. In 1819 it listed only thirteen female midwives, whereas the number of man-midwives had risen to forty-two. Scholten (1985: 32).

65. W. Tyler Smith (1849: 501).

66. In Latin, "Obstetrix" meant midwife (specifically a female midwife) as early as the second century B.C.E. Personal communication, William S. Bonds, professor of Classical Studies, University of South Sewanee, Tennessee, 16 September 1998.

67. Rongy (1937: 98).

68. Householder (1974: 429).

69. J. F. Osiander (1829: 169). Coincidentally, slow labor is now considered unhealthy. If a woman labors for "too long" in contemporary hospital settings, her chances of having induced labor or a cesarean section are greatly increased. See Anders (1993).

70. "Würde eine Frauen allein ohne Beistand gebären, so würde sie nicht stehen oder sitzend gebären. Sie würde von der Natur angehalten, ein weiches Lager zu bereiten oder aufzusuchen und dadurch selbst die Schonung des Mittelfleisches bewerk-

stelligen. Daher ist das Gebären auf dem Stuhle regelwidrig und ganz zu verwerfen, denn wenn bei dieser Art zu gebären der Damm nicht einreißt, so ist es nicht der Kunst der Hebamme, sondern dem natürlichen Gange der Sache zuschreiben. Es ist überhaupt eine irrige Meinung, daß die Gebärende auf dem Stuhl besser sich halte und dadurch leichter und geschwinder gebären könne. Alles was dabei gewonnen wird, ist, daß das Bettwerk nicht so sehr verschmutzt und verdorben wird und aus dieser Ursache findet die Abschaffung des Gebärstuhles vielen Widerstand." Schweighäuser (1817: 190).

71. "Der Gebärstuhl ist nichts andres als ein Schutzmittel gegen die Verunreinigung des Bettzeugs, und deshalb ist dieser vor allem bei unbemittelten und geizigen Frauen beliebt. Der Mehrzahl der Gebärenden verwirft den Gebärstuhl, da ihnen vor den Plackereien beim Aufschlagen, dem Draufliegen und den vielen anderen Umständlichkeiten und Unbequemlichkeiten graut." J. F. Osiander (1829: 171).

72. "Meine Abneigung gegen den Stuhl für die Privatpraxis ist daraus entstanden, daß ich oft Gelegenheit gehabt habe, die schlechte Beschaffenheit, die willkürlichen Abänderungen und damit Verunstaltungen der Gebärstuhl die Hebammen kennenzulernen und leider oft gewahlt zy werden, daß eine solche unbehilfliche Maschine, an der das Blut und die Schweiß vom Virtage noch klebt, nicht nur zum Entbinden widrig sondern auch dem Geburtshelfer mehr hinderlich als förderlich ist." F. B. Osiander (1825: 402).

73. Cassar (1973: 60).

74. "das größte Verdienst in der Verbannen des Gebärstuhl aus Gebärstuben und gebärstalten zu." Quoted in Fasbender (1906: 269).

75. Henrich Lakämper-Lührs, Stadtmuseum Güntersloh, letter to author, 28 July 1992.

76. Speert (1973: Fig. 9.13).

77. O'Dowd and Philipp (1994: 20–21).

78. O'Dowd and Philipp (1994: 174).

Contest and Compromise:
The Debate over the Philosophy of Birth, the Return of the Birth Chair, and the Struggle for Ownership

The drastic changes in the philosophy of birth that occurred the nineteenth century culminated in thought and deed in the twentieth. In response, the cultural construction of birth was composed of a definition of birth as a pathological event, and the practice was increasingly characterized by prescribed medical procedures and clinical personnel. Although such a shift in philosophy did consolidate the authority of medicine to define birth and thus to drive and determine appropriate procedures and practices, the medical philosophy remained an unquestioned construction only until the middle years of the century.

By the 1950s, changes in society and, in association, alterations in the birth process, medicine, and women, began a process of questioning this medical approach to practice. When it became apparent that questioning these practices resulted in little change, a limited faction of society began to openly discuss and debate the underlying philosophy. In this context of debate, the authority to define birth did not remain solely in the hands of professional medicine. Practices began to reflect not just the prevailing philosophy of medicine, but also an alternative and diametrically opposed definition of birth.

As with earlier periods, studying the practices of birth and its associated artifacts in the twentieth century elucidates the dynamics of this debate and the beliefs of all parturients and practitioners. In the twentieth century there are multiple artifacts, some of which are "items" such as the location of delivery, the secondary written histories of birth, the tests and procedures employed by professional obstetrics, as well as the external materials manufactured or modified for use in delivery such as birth chairs, delivery tables, the family bed, and other such devices.

Interviews with practicing midwives, doctors, and delivering women and the study of the social, political, and economic contexts of this century reveal a material history of contemporary birth that is separate from a discussion of a systematic advancement of techniques, procedures, and medical discoveries. Rather, with two functioning philosophies of birth, it becomes an exciting area of debate where the power of attitude is most palatable. Through the artifacts, we can see the importance of a philosophy in shaping practice and the multifaceted ways in which a cultural construction of birth is formed.

Hospitals, the Twilight Sleep, and Scientific Childbirth

As an artifact of birth, the physical location of delivery has much to reveal about the contemporary history of birth. For example, the move from home to hospital for delivery at the turn of the century finalized the perception of birth as a medical emergency and cemented an understanding of effective practice requiring not only medical procedures, but a medical locale as well. Maternity hospitals, or lying-in centers, were first used by the indigent population of major cities. Here, poor women were delivered in exchange for their use as test cases and models for medical students. However, birth in hospitals among women who were not offering themselves as test cases, but as paying customers, rose radically following the introduction of anesthesia, most particularly in its apex, the "twilight sleep."[1] This method, introduced by Bernhard Krönig in Germany in 1899, used a combination of morphine and scopolamine and caused an amnesiac and unconscious state. Regarded as a blessing to women because it removed all pain and erased most memory of the birth process, women began using hospitals with increasingly regularity to gain access to this procedure.

Like the changes brought about by developments of medical technique such as forceps, the use of anesthesia affected the process and practice of birth significantly. Its use drew pregnant women to hospitals and encouraged hospitals' growing popularity. It also widened the pool of medical personnel "required" for an effective birth. The use of anesthesia dramatically altered the postures for delivery, in that an unconscious woman made any manner of delivery but a recumbent, often restrained, position impossible. Its use also increased the portrayal of women as too ineffective to manage the process alone.

This anesthetized approach to delivery is clearly seen in the delivery devices of the day. Delivery in hospitals took place in operating rooms, or "theaters," on flat tables or hospital gurneys that included arm straps and sometimes foot straps. Such additions and designs suggest the growing attitude that women needed to be controlled and contained during this event. An example is an official "delivery table" from the Sloane Maternity Hospital in New York City (c. 1910). The only thing that separates this device from an operating table is a crank system that would raise the upper portion of the table about ten inches, which would slightly elevate the head of the delivering woman (Figure 3.1). Because it so closely resembled an operating table, this item clearly closed all remaining distance between birth as natural and birth as an event that required intervention.

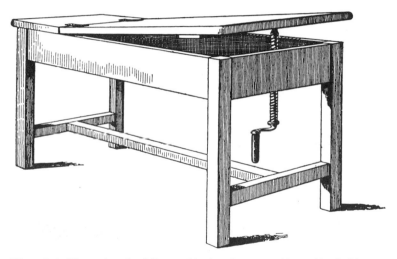

Figure 3.1. Illustration of a delivery table, American, c. 1910, used in the Sloane Maternity Hospital, New York City. From Harold Speert's Iconographia Gyniatrica *(1973). Reprinted by permission.*

With a well-defined philosophy of birth, an appropriate physical space, and new tools, medicine dictated practices and established acceptable regimens for delivery. In accordance with such a philosophy and as practiced in a standard, "normal" birth, the woman would lie "throughout the second stage, in a perfectly natural, comfortable, and non-fatiguing position which she cannot change, even when only incompletely narcotized."[2] Thus, by

1926 a narcotized and restricted state was considered the natural and normal one for birth. This statement fully reflects the attitude of professional medicine toward women and birth-giving in the early twentieth century. Under this new philosophy of birth, all a woman had to do was, "keep her spirits up, and adhere strictly to the rules of her medical advisor."[3] The popularity of such an unconscious state indicated clearly that medical professionals felt no birth could be successfully accomplished without assistance and certainly on no device other than an elevated, flat surface. It is equally clear that the woman's role was considered insignificant in the birth act, that birth was an event in which women were, ironically, unqualified to participate.

Anesthesia and birth in a hospital setting ideologically changed the process of birth as well. While professional medicine advocated these new approaches to birth as a blessing to women, there was simultaneously a growing belief that the advocacy of doctors and public health officials would dispel the notion that hospitals were unclean charity wards. Medical professionals believed that as hospital use grew popular—enhanced by the liberal application of anesthesia—the low birth rate among the more "desirable" upper classes would rise and thereby increase the economic rewards of obstetrics. The cultivation of a medical perception of birth had had a double-edged effect for medicine. It had enhanced physicians' control and cornered the market for obstetricians, but it had perhaps also driven down the birth rate among upper-class (paying) clientele. As J. P. Mcvoy stated in 1938, the use of anesthesia would remove women's fear of labor to the extent that more children would be "born in the white collar and professional groups where at present the [low] birth rate is causing grave alarm."[4] Whether hospitals and anesthesia actually provided better care was not important (a 1912 study by Johns Hopkins Hospital indicated the opposite); what mattered was that they were believed to do so by society. In effect, doctors used anesthesia as a means to further their control over birth and possibly increase the number of births in hospitals.[5] In fact, in the United States births in hospitals rapidly increased from 36.9 percent of all births in 1935 to 99.4 percent in 1970.[6]

The preeminence of such a philosophy shaped practice to the extent that birth became a medical event where doctors acted upon a woman's body to achieve delivery. Birth was accomplished in an exaggerated lithotomy position, where the woman was placed on a delivery table flat on her back with her feet and legs raised high above her hips. The delivery artifacts of the time clear-

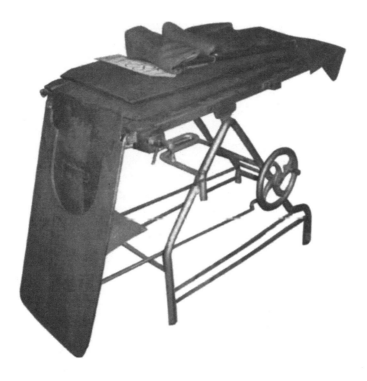

Figure 3.2. Obstetric table, English, c. 1930–1955, now in the collection of The National Museum of Science and Industry, London. When assembled, the woman labored in a horizontal position, either over a circular opening or, with the placement of the table insertion, over a closed opening. Photograph by author.

ly portray such an approach. Beginning as tables like the one used in the Sloane Hospital (see Figure 3.1), like birth chairs, these artifacts were elaborated and technologically altered to "enhance" their usefulness and their image. They quickly became delivery stretchers or surgical tables with numerous innovations. One such table used from 1930 until the late 1940s has no adjustable back to elevate the head or upper back of the laboring woman (Figure 3.2). The table has stirrups attachments, and the woman would slide down to the bottom, where a flat attachment would lengthen the table. This device has a semicircular cutout similar to the Güntersloh table; the woman would give birth over this opening with her feet in the stirrups, presumably in the narcotized and helpless state that was regarded as normal.

The effect of such a mentality and the associated posture is illustrated in the following account of birth from 1937:

Arriving [at the hospital] she is immediately given the benefit of one of the modern analgesics or pain-killers. Soon she is in a dreamy, half-conscious state . . . she knows nothing about being taken to a spotlessly clean delivery room, placed on a sterile table, draped with sterile sheets, neither does she see her attendants, the doctor and nurses, garbed for her protection in sterile white gowns and gloves, nor the shiny boiled instruments and antiseptic solutions. She does not hear the cry of her baby when first he feels the chill of this cold world, or see the care with which the doctor repairs such laceration as may have occurred. . . . Finally, she awakes in smiles, a mother with no recollection of having become one.7

This narcotized, highly invasive approach to birth was the norm for the first half of the twentieth century. This approach systematically developed into such a routinized regimen that any question or alteration to the practice was not tolerated. By the 1940s, delivery was not something a woman did in concert with nature. Rather, birth was something that was done to her—a crisis situation from which she needed to be rescued.

The early years of the twentieth century were characterized by a consolidation of the medical redefinition of birth with attendant locale and practice, a distinct shift in the cultural construction of birth, and a concerted effort to eliminate all practices of birth associated with uninformed, and possible unhygienic, midwives. However, these years also brought the publication of secondary texts that rewrote the history of birth to fit this understanding. These texts, the majority of which were written by medical professionals, recount the history of birth as chronological and evolutionary and operated under the belief that medicine "developed from its crudest, most primitive form into its modern, Western, highly sophisticated state. All that was most effective was retained during this evolutionary ascent, while discarded and obsolete ideas drifted downward and were preserved in the lower levels."8 The history of birth was portrayed as a process that improved with time, became more effective with medical progress, and changed due to advances in the techniques and profession of medical science, the growth in the understanding of anatomy and physiology, the increase in the number of trained obstetricians, and the dismissal of ignorant midwives.

These histories are significant in that they created a male genealogy for all of obstetrical history. They glorified the later obstetrical practitioners for freeing medicine from the burdens of antiquated midwifery practices. However, these obstetrical histories are also ironic. While giving muted credit to early writers such as Rueff, Rösslin, and Guillimeau, they fail to mention that these writers directed their works to practicing midwives, not physicians, and that these writers rarely, if ever, attended births except in life-or-death situations. W. Tyler Smith went very far in his revision of birth history, crediting only William Harvey, Peter Chamberlain, and William Hunter as the "fathers of obstetrics."[9] This view was staunchly founded on the premise of birth as pathology and the ineffective, often meddlesome nature of those nonmedical personnel from whom birth had been saved— women and midwives. According to such accounts, it was only due to the entrance of men into this field that women were saved from pain, dismemberment, and death. It was not until the 1970s that new work on the history of birth began to undo the created histories of this period. These newer works addressed the medical establishment of the nineteenth century and the reinterpretation of medicine, female health, and birth.[10]

An additional product of these secondary texts was occasional academic, although not clinical, interest in birth chairs. As other practices associated with premedicalized birth, birth chairs were regarded in these early histories as elements of the poor, the backward, and the unenlightened. However, birth chairs were equally seen as a curiosity that provided further evidence of the advances of medical science.[11] The efforts of C. J. S. Thompson (1862–1943) at the Wellcome Institute in London are an example of this. Thompson was interested in birth chairs and commissioned the construction of four birth chairs in the workshop at the institute. However, his perspective was historical, and he discussed birth chairs only as an element of past and outdated practices of delivery. Thompson's chairs were reconstructions of descriptions and sketches from historical texts and were used only as display items.[12]

Concurrent with Thompson's work at the Wellcome Institute, Dr. Albert King and Dr. James Markoe at the Lying-In Hospital in New York City wrote articles briefly surveying the history of birth postures, including a section on birth chairs. Markoe later built and actually tested two birth chairs at the Lying-In Hospital (Figure 3.3). Although he used his chairs at the hospital among the charitable cases and kept statistics of their successes, he still insisted that his chairs were "in no way intended as a delivery table."[13] He believed that more research and design elaboration would be necessary to

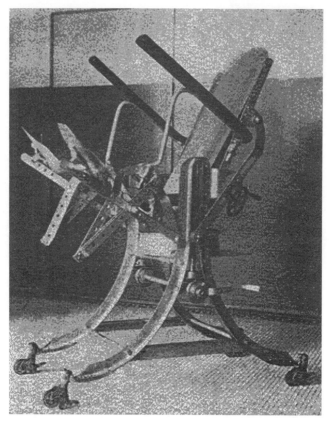

Figure 3.3. A birth chair constructed and tested by James Markoe at the Lying-In Hospital in New York City, c. 1915. From the Bulletin of the Lying-in Hospital *(1915).*

make his chairs acceptable as birth tools. In comparison to earlier successful birth chairs, the Markoe chairs were actually highly elaborate and offered more innovations than any previous chair. The influence of the concept of birth as an event that required extensive resources and great levels of intervention was so pervasive that Markoe doubted the effectiveness of his birth chair in delivery without even more adaptations.

Birth Chairs as Exam Tables

As we have seen with the "Voltaire Chairs" of the late nineteenth century, the designs of these rejected, ridiculed, and dismissed artifacts of birth were

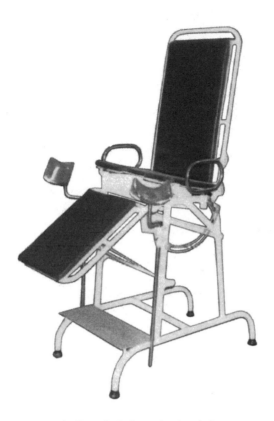

Figure 3.4. Gynecological examination chair,
Germany, c. 1925–1935, in the collection of The
National Museum of Science and Industry, London.
Photograph by author.

co-opted by the new field of gynecology, which dealt with the "diseases" of women. This borrowing of style and design from condemned items of birth for use in advocated items of professional medicine was furthered in the early twentieth century, as seen in the growth of manufacturing and marketing of special obstetrical/gynecological chairs. Such items are significant in that they harken back to the design of birth chairs and because of what their existence means. As chairs designed specifically for gynecological exams, they indicate that doctors had indeed arrived as legitimate and socially acceptable practitioners of birth. These items were important for their ironic borrowing of design. However, they also made clear the redefinition of not only birth, but women's health in general, where special chairs were required to care for the particular issues of women's health then gaining attention. These chairs appear to be birth chairs and lack only the defining characteristic, the semi-circular opening in the seat. With even higher seats, approximately thirty inches from the ground, these chairs possess modified ratchet backs, stirrups or knee braces instead of footrests, and small drawers under the seat for tool storage. They are similar in appearance to a child's high chair. One German gynecological chair (c. 1925) features an equipment tray, folding knee braces, hand-holds, and a back that can be lowered to accommodate a full lithotomy position (Figure 3.4).

Motherhood under the Microscope

As noted, medical professionals nurtured the perception that motherhood was an area that women were largely unqualified to participate in without medical control and direction. Professionals likewise made scientific many other aspects of women's lives, exerting their control and authority in all manners of things.[14] This interpretation is borne out in the study of artifacts as well. Manufacturers marketed medically advocated baby bottles (with instructions on how to feed a child), hygienic diapers (with instructions on how to change and clothe a child), prepared baby food (with instructions on how to feed a child), and countless other items that were designed for proper and scientific childrearing. Publishers followed with manuals and instructional guides written by doctors to help usher a woman through pregnancy, birth, and motherhood. Hospitals, government agencies, and doctors advocated special programs, classes, and lectures designed to teach a woman how to manage and understand these processes. For example, in 1918 authorities in Ontario opened ten centers to hold workshops and lectures to teach women how to bathe, feed, diaper, and attend to their children in the appropriate and now scientific fashion.[15]

There was an occasional article or doctor who presented evidence against the accepted postures and protocols of birth, instead advocating the more physiologically sound and traditional approach to birth. However, the medical cultural construction of birth was deeply entrenched, and regardless of this "fringe" interest, birth practices remained unaltered because they reflected the medical philosophy. As Forest Howard pointed out in "The Physiologic Position for Delivery," any study or reevaluation of upright birth, even in a hospital delivery room, would be difficult.[16] The researcher would first have to address the negativity of the whole idea and counter questions about his suspected challenge to the prevailing medical philosophy. Until society changed its views about birth, there could be no changes in the practice of birth. Convinced of the physiological benefits of upright labor and delivery as safer for women, Howard designed an upright delivery device as an alternative to the operating table for delivery. Although he did not question the pathological definition of birth or even the preferred location for delivery, he was confronted with the power of the medical hegemony over birth and the summary dismissal of his designs. He stated, "Our present mores as a group are such that conservative thinking in this respect is regarded as being quite radical, and my table has not been allowed in any of the nearby hospitals. Little by little I would hope to convince my colleagues of the worthwhileness of this project. The patients are not hard to convince."[17]

Any practice of birth that strayed from the regimented protocol of doctor-attended birth in a clinical surrounding and the subsequent adherence to doctor-mandated childrearing was considered dated, primitive, dangerous, radical, and highly unacceptable. Birth chairs or any alternative delivery device were particularly offensive. However, the changes that Howard deemed necessary to open a dialogue about the ideology of birth and to affect birth practices began to appear by midcentury. The widespread, common experiences of women due to the surge in the birth rate from the mid-1940s to the early 1960s, referred to as "the baby boom," and the massive move to the suburbs nurtured an increase in contact and community among women, finally creating a context in which the topic of birth was again considered acceptable for discourse.

The Rise of Questioning and Alternatives in Birth

As women discussed birth, in general, and the actual details of the delivery process, they questioned the standard medical approach to childbirth. This dialogue originally dealt only with the physical treatment of the mother and did not question the actual conceptualization of birth as a crisis event. Eventually, the undercurrent of displeasure and doubt about the treatment of women during birth led to questions about the intrinsic perception of birth itself.

The public debate over the use of interventionist practices and the prevailing appraisal of birth as a crisis situation began slowly, starting with the appearance of articles in the *Ladies Home Journal* and other similar publications. Peter Briggs's "Faulty Care and Infant Deaths" (1955) and particularly Gladys Shultz's "Cruelty in Maternity Wards" (1958) generated tremendous reader response that detailed the treatment or mistreatment of women laboring in hospitals.[18] Readers described being strapped down and left alone for hours, being denied any liquids, and having their requests and appeals ignored. Defenders of these "treatments" and of the prevailing philosophy stated that women needed to be strapped down "to prevent contamination of the sterile field" and that "many women are spoiled, hysterical and full of fears; . . . the memory of a childbirth experience is unreliable because of anesthetic drugs; [and] there is simply not enough hospital and medical staff to give women the kind of care they seem to demand."[19]

If not yet the philosophy of society as a whole, the dialogue among women stimulated by articles like Shultz's and the questions surrounding the treatment soon expanded to include the use of drugs and forceps, induction of labor, separation of mother from child, and the arbitrary regimen of hospitals. Finally, this dialogue came to include the attitude toward birth as pathological and women in childbirth as equivalent to malfunctioning machines (Figure 3.5).[20] Questions arose as to whether hospitals really were the best atmosphere for delivery and whether such regimented treatments were truly the best way to practice birth. A growing number of observers argued that birth injuries and maternal mortality were, in fact, actually greater in hospitals precisely because of this interference with the normal birth process.[21] These concerns were supported by the statistics. Home midwifery services of the 1940s and 1950s, like the Maternity Center of New York and the Frontier Nursing Service of Kentucky, had lower infant and maternal mortality rates than most hospitals and significantly lower incidents of iatrogenic (doctor-caused) complications and nosocomial (hospital-caused) infections.[22]

An important product of this growing dialogue was Marjorie Karmel's 1959 book, *Thank you, Dr. Lamaze,* which detailed the standard birth process in contrast to the more natural approach she had experienced in France. Bolstered by information about the growing popularity in Europe of methods of birth like *Accouchement Sans Douleur* (the Lamaze method) and the methods of Grantly Dick-Read and Frederick Leboyer, women sought to reduce unnecessary intervention in their deliveries and to defeat patronizing

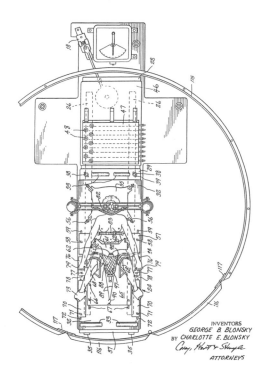

Figure 3.5. Perhaps the greatest evidence of the perception of delivering women as malfunctioning machines and the advocacy of the use of mechanized tools of birth is captured in an American invention from the early 1960s. Although never widely used, the inventors advocated strapping down the "under-equipped woman" and spinning her to propel the infant through the birth canal. George D. Blonsky et al., "Apparatus for Facilitating the Birth of a Child by Centrifugal Force," U.S. patent number 3,216,423, granted 9 November 1965.

attitudes of professional medicine captured in comments like, "Don't worry, Honey. All you have to do is have the baby, I'll do the rest."[23] Instead, advocates of natural childbirth sought a return of attitudes like those of Dr. Fernand Lamaze, who told Marjorie Karmel, "You have your baby yourself, I am only there to assist you."[24] It was with this debate that a movement for alternative birth began, a movement that original questioned the approaches to birth and soon realized the necessity of redefining the prevailing philosophy of birth to reshape the practices of delivery.

During the 1960s and 1970s, other movements and ideas fostered and encouraged the alternative birth movement. In the United States, social movements like the protests against the Vietnam War and for civil rights nurtured a general skepticism toward organizations, professionals, and "the establishment." Women's rights and feminism further contributed to a questioning of the professional medical agenda and particularly of women's health issues. Feminists argued that medicine needed to be demystified and women's lives demedicalized, particularly citing the belief that pregnancy and childbirth were normal, nondisease states.[25] This movement gained momentum with the popularity of alternative lifestyles at places like The Farm in Tennessee and the growing consciousness and emphasis on experiencing and appreciating nature.[26] Ina May Gaskin, cofounder of The Farm, published *Spiritual Midwifery,* a splendid example of the mentality, approach, and redefinition of birth that alternative movements hoped to bring about.

Scandals like that surrounding thalidomide, a morning-sickness drug that resulted in serious birth deformities, shook physicians and pharmaceutical companies and undermined the unwavering trust previously paid to them by the public. In addition, the development of forms of socialized medicine in postwar western Europe also effectively questioned the context for highly invasive approaches to birth. As indicated by the growing number of medical malpractice suits, the authority of the medical profession was no longer beyond question.[27] Although certainly still an issue, many of the societal contexts (for example, financial rewards and competition for clientele) that allowed the interpretation of birth as exclusively pathological had been removed in western European countries. The struggle over the philosophy and practice of birth and the need to develop a material history to navigate the meaning and significance of this alternative birth movement became an increasingly American phenomenon.[28]

The Alternative Birth Movement

Encompassing a wide variety of natural, alternative, and noninterventionist practices, the movement for alternative birth placed value on the mother's role and strove for practices that worked in concert with birth, rather than those that attempted to dictate and manipulate it. The designation "alternative birth movement" represented the many organizations that advocated and practiced any method of childbirth other than conventional hospital labor and delivery. In *Alternative Birth: The Complete Guide,* Carl Jones described this movement as "a philosophy of childbirth in which labor and birth are viewed as a natural and normal process, rather than as an illness or a clinical procedure."[29] This movement looked to traditional practices and the growing trend toward self-care for models and questioned the conventional practice of delivery, the use of highly invasive techniques, and the pervasive attitude of pregnancy and birth as a crisis in desperate need of management. The alternative birth movement strove to return childbirth to the family and to nature. It emphasized a holistic approach, often symbolized by the return of birth to the home and family bed, where birth could the focal point of a family-centered event rather than a medical event—a time of celebration and not of "coming down to death's door."

In attempting to alter practice, the alternative birth movement moved to contest the hegemony of professional medicine and challenge and redefine all aspects of the medical philosophy.[30] For this reason, the contemporary struggle between alternative birth practices and professional obstetrics in the United States proves fundamental to the discussion of the power that a prevailing philosophy exercises over the actual practice of birth and the utility of studying these practices to clarify and identify the whole cultural construction of birth.

Artifacts of birth, both those of professional medicine and those of the alternative birth movement, again illustrate the ideological issues that are at stake as well as the antagonists' agendas as they negotiate and interpret the practices of birth. Birth chairs, delivery beds, adapted materials of the home, and numerous other manufactured alternative delivery devices reveal information about the desire to recreate an alternative, woman-driven, back-to-nature approach to delivery and the medical-centered understanding of the process. As noted above, the chosen location for delivery, such as delivery rooms, labor-delivery-recovery rooms, birth centers, and the home, act as artifacts of birth and similarly reveal information about not only the practice of birth, but the ideology behind it.

In the United States, the challenge of the prevailing medical philosophy of birth is illustrated by the creation of birth centers, where birth could be practiced as it reflected the alternative philosophy.[31] For example, in 1976 the Maternity Center of New York City expanded its services by establishing an area within the center where it could offer an experience separate from the "interference" of hospitals. In this area, a double bed, homelike decor, and other nonmedical items were present, thus creating the image of birth as natural and nonmedical. The Bryn Mawr Birth Center in Bryn Mawr,

Pennsylvania (founded in 1980), and Women Care, Inc., in Monett, Missouri (founded in 1981), offered similar settings that were separate from the hospital ideology and practice.[32] In these centers, it was possible to practice birth in concert with a natural philosophy and as if the birth was merely an extension of home life because the artifacts of the medical philosophy and the medical practice were absent. Alternative birth centers and alternative practitioners both cultivated a nonmedical understanding and encouraged laboring women to experiment with different postures and forms of delivery. These alternative practices allowed mothers to design and direct their own experiences and determine for themselves what would make them most comfortable, at ease, and successful in the process.

By 1987, 240 free-standing birth centers had been established in the United States.[33] Simultaneously, the attendance of midwives and nurse-midwives instead of doctors in birth centers and at home rose dramatically. In 1975, certified nurse-midwives were responsible for 19,685 of the 4,144,198 (0.4 percent) recorded births in the United States. By 1989, they were responsible for 122,892 of the 4,040,958 (3 percent) recorded births, and by 1996, this figure had risen to approximately 6 percent.[34] Also, midwives practicing without certification or licensing, which is unavailable in many states and illegal in many others, attended countless births.[35] As artifacts, these centers reveal how a more natural understanding of birth allows for a more natural practice of delivery.

Birth centers continue to provide contradictory examples of the power of belief to direct practice.[36] As Dr. Marsden G. Wagner, the former European director of maternal and child health of the World Health Organization, made clear, "Every single country in the European region with prenatal and infant-mortality rates lower than the United States uses midwives as the principal and only birth attendant for at least 70 percent of all births."[37] Birth-center statistics stood as clear examples of the efficiency of certified nurse-midwives and of the alternative birth movement. However, among physicians, ideology proved stronger than statistics. By 1987, the New Jersey Obstetrics and Gynecology Society had repeatedly affirmed that birth centers "are not in the best interest of the safety and care of obstetrics and gynecology patients."[38] Regardless of their success rates, because they were uncondoned by the medical philosophy, birth centers remained a fringe element.

As a result of this growing movement for natural birth, numerous alternative journals and alternative birth retailers offered and advocated birthing

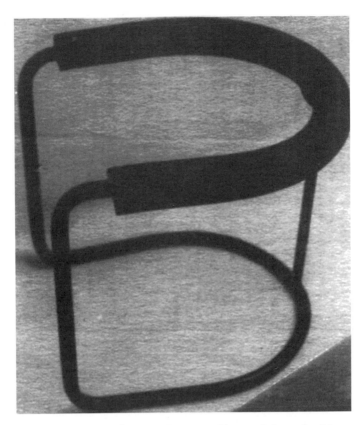

Figure 3.6. "deBy Birth Support," c. 1992. Photograph from advertising materials, deBy Birth Supports, Barrington, New Hampshire.

devices.[39] These items reflect an atmosphere of experimentation, an unregimented approach to delivery, and an understanding of the choices and preferences of the delivering woman as paramount. Some manufactures advocated the soothing effects of being born into this world in a watery environment similar to the amniotic sack. Birth in water, such as in tubs, swimming pools, inflatable delivery pools, or among dolphins, was one delivery alternative. Others alternative items included inflatable balls for supporting squatting positions during labor and delivery, stools, delivery pans, and delivery hammocks.[40]

An example of an artifact reflective of this alternative, noninterventionist, natural philosophy of birth is the deBy Birth Support (Figure 3.6). Designed by an Amsterdam midwife, it is a solid metal frame with sponge-rubber padding along the top for comfort and gripping. It allows the laboring and delivering woman to support herself in a squatting position, while allowing access to the birth canal and to the back for massage and support. Additionally, women can sit on it and use it as a birth stool. Its size and weight make transportation between deliveries easy. Marketed by Moonflower Birthing Supply and other sources, it is a popular item among alternative birth centers and practicing midwives.[41]

The artifacts that were most telling of the intent, message, and philosophy of the movement was the rediscovery and reintroduction of the birth chair as a viable device for labor and delivery, as seen in such items as the deBy device and in contemporary handbuilt birth chairs and stools. Birth chairs found new popularity for the utility of their design and use and for the message or image they portrayed—a return to the "golden age" of midwifery, with a women-centered, natural, event-drive approach to birth.

Although ripe with imagery, the use of birth chairs and stools in such alternative surroundings is limited to those centers that have handmade birth chairs or stools or have purchased one of the few available low-cost stools produced and marketed by companies targeted to home births and alternative centers. An example is a birth stool in use at the Maternity

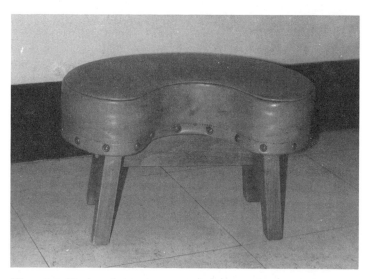

Figure 3.7. Birth stool, American, c. 1985, in use at the Maternity Center in New York City. Constructed and marketed in the 1980s by The Family Life Center of Albany, New York. Photograph by author.

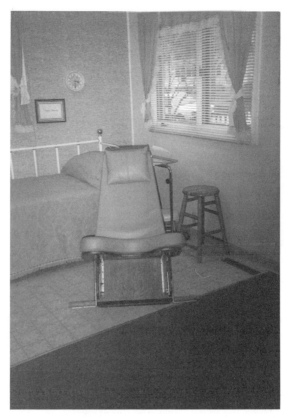

Figure 3.8. Handmade birth chair, American, 1990, in use at Woman Care, Inc., Monett, Missouri. Photograph courtesy of Lessa Ginther, Woman Care, Inc.

Center in New York City (Figure 3.7). Constructed and marketed by The Family Life Center of Albany, New York (no longer in business), this is a semicircular stool with a seat height of ten inches. It offers the characteristic semicircular, cutout seat, which is upholstered in vinyl. This stool allows for an upright posture, access for the midwife or other attendants to the birth canal and to the woman for massage and support, and freedom of movement for the mother. According to the director of the Maternity Center, this stool is often used by the midwife when the mother chooses other postures for delivery, including standing in the shower area at the center, sitting on the edge of the double bed, or other selected positions.[42]

Handmade birth chairs and stools that capture the imagery of the alternative birth movement and that harken back to the traditional era of birth are also in use at other alternative birth centers and among lay midwives.[43] The birth center Woman Care, Inc., of Monett, Missouri, has a 90-percent use rate for its birth chairs. Their chairs, one for in-center use and one for in-home delivery, were designed and built by the center director's husband in 1990 based on historic designs and from observation of women delivering at the center.[44] Both chairs are lightweight and similar in design to beach chairs, with a semicircular seat opening that is low enough to the ground to allow for bracing by the mother. The in-center chair (Figure 3.8) has a high back that can be placed at various angles from semirecumbent to completely upright. There are no arms, although hand-holds are attached to the seat for bracing and support, and the back is supported by a brace. The chair folds for transportation.

Although not used by all clientele, birth chairs find popularity in the imagery that their presence conveys even in the exceptional birthing center located in a hospital. The Pennsylvania Hospital's Birthing Suite owns such an example. In 1986, after experiencing the birth of his son, a father designed, built, and donated a birth chair to the hospital (Figure 3.9). Based on suggestions from midwives and personal observation, this chair is strikingly similar in design and dimensions of older birth chairs, although no historical research was done.[45] This chair is approximately forty inches high at its back and has a semicircular seat opening approximately seventeen inches from the ground. The chair lacks arms or hand-holds and is upholstered in oilcloth with a nursery motif. According to the director of the Birthing Suite, this chair is often used by women during labor and delivery, although many do not choose the device unless they are offered it, even though it stands in the birth room. The director believes that this is because, although it is a birth center, in the hospital setting his patients still require permission to act in a manner separate from the way they have been conditioned to view birth.[46] Most birth chairs used in home births and in birth centers are not the products of major medical manufacturing companies, but are products of alternative birth companies and local members of the community, thus reflecting the philosophy of the movement.

Birth chairs and stools, as well as the other artifacts of delivery, are significant not only for the style of labor and delivery they suggest and advocate, but for their role as tangible signs of the direct challenge to the medicalized philosophy of birth and its associated practices. Regardless of level

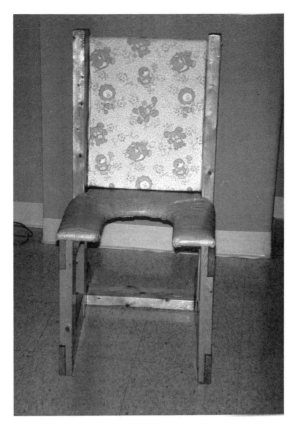

Figure 3.9. Handmade birth chair, American, 1986, in use in the Birthing Suite of the Pennsylvania Hospital, Philadelphia. Photograph by author.

of use, the presence of birth chairs in these nonhospital settings signaled a change from the philosophy and practice of official obstetrics to alternative practices that reflect a woman-centered, physiology-based, and natural/traditional approach to the process. They function as symbols for the philosophy of the movement where birth was regarded as a natural, nonmedical event. For example, the Schlosser-Alberti Company (no longer in business) advertised their birth chair as "reflective of the concept of natural delivery."[47]

Another important aspect of these alternative birth centers and the alternative movement, in general, was their argument for an educated and informed approach to pregnancy and birth with an emphasis on a natural, noninterventionist labor and delivery and a willingness to try new and alternative approaches. This education was achieved through childbirth classes, which were first offered at places like the local YWCA, the alternative centers, and local churches and synagogues. These classes taught women and their partners what to expect in pregnancy and birth, in some way attempting to "re-educate" them, and provided information about their many options for the actual delivery. A related book industry grew rapidly, including instruction manuals for home birth, well-pregnancy guides, and histories of the alternative movement.[48] Aside from the large number of works from the popular presses, there was also a burgeoning dialogue within the alternative movement that included small-press books, support groups, and telephone networks. In the 1970s and early 1980s, alternative birth also gained popularity as a topic in the mainstream press, with hundreds of articles concerning alternative approaches to birth and the use of birth chairs running in major newspapers like the *Los Angeles Times, New York Times,* and *Washington Post* and on wire services like the Associated Press and United Press International.[49] The resulting communication, publications, and education expanded the alternative birth movement to a larger sector of the general public. As a result, societal attitudes about birth began to slightly change. Women now expected doctors to adhere to their wishes and, if this was not possible, to consult them and elicit approval or permission before performing any procedure.

For example, when searching for a doctor during her first pregnancy, Melanie L. of Bloomington, Indiana, compiled a list of twenty questions. She asked and required answers to such questions as "What is the policy on routine intervention? What is the cesarean rate in the practice, for the doctor, in the hospital? How many mothers receive pitocin to stimulate labor? Do you have time limits for any stage of labor? If so, what are they?" Melanie educated herself and planned carefully for any contingency, requiring complete control of the process and of any decisions that were to be made. Several months later, Melanie was the only one in her six-member Lamaze class who delivered vaginally.[50]

Compromise and Consolidation

In addition to the alternative birth movement's challenge of the profession's modus operandi, by the early 1980s professional obstetrics was being confronted with a sagging birth rate that limited available profits, an increasing frequency of medical malpractice suits, and soaring insurance rates.[51] The assaults on physicians provided the impetus to cultivate an even more medical philosophy of birth, while attempting to attract more clients without alienating them. Professional obstetrics created and enhanced approaches to birth that both compromised with alternative ideology and consolidated the medical approach. The artifacts of medical birth reveal this clearly. Doctors developed and implemented extensive prenatal tests and procedures, "alternative" or nondelivery room settings for birth, new tools for delivery, and legal means to reassert their authority in the birthing process.

In an effort to keep birth in hospitals and to compete with other hospitals for the declining number of births, professional medicine responded with its own "alternative" version. To this end, professional obstetrics introduced hospital-based alternative birth centers and labor-delivery-recovery rooms, where the woman remained throughout her hospital stay. These venues implemented more "homey" decor with patterned wallpaper, wooden furniture, private baths, rocking chairs, and, significantly, double beds in the alternative birth centers and delivery beds in the labor-delivery-recovery rooms. These beds provided a variety of positions so that a woman could remain in the same room throughout the birth process, instead of being moved from a labor room to a delivery room to a recovery room to a hospital room.[52] Examples include the Women's Pavilion at the Baptist Hospital in Nashville, Tennessee (created in 1981), and the Birthing Suite at the Pennsylvania Hospital in Philadelphia (created in 1983).[53]

Compromises in the conventional hospital practice of birth allowed some different approaches to labor, such as reducing or not using drugs during labor, an increase in the woman's freedom of movement and posture during labor (although a modified lithotomy position was still advocated and encouraged during the actual delivery), attendance of the father and perhaps other family members, and even a nurse-midwife as long as there was a doctor in attendance. Like the alternative centers, area hospitals also began routinely providing childbirth education classes, although for a fee. However, these classes concentrated more on teaching women what to expect from hospital protocol and providing the basics in child care, while concentrating less on the options women had in actual delivery.[54]

Such compromise was essential to professional obstetrics because research indicated that women represented sixty percent of all hospital business and made up to eighty-five percent of all medical decisions in a family.[55] As

Jackie Reinhardt, a Beverly Hills hospital marketing consultant, stated, "Women's services are really hot in the health-care field, and obstetrics is that critical area when you enter that market and where you can cross-sell once you get this woman."[56] In 1987, a marketing vice-president at Valley Presbyterian in Los Angeles reiterated this idea, "When we put our program together, we felt that if a woman delivered here, she would bring her baby here. That would be the linkage. And along with that child would come the father and whoever else was in the family."[57] This sounds very similar to Dr. Channing's advice from 1820: "Women seldom forget a practitioner who has conducted them tenderly and safely through parturition. . . . It is principally on this account that the practice of midwifery becomes desirable to physicians. It is this which insures to the permancy [sic] and security of all their other business."[58]

This show of compromise, however, was primarily limited to the user-friendly decor of hospital rooms and subtle alterations in the location of the actual delivery, which were the easiest to create, the most immediately visible, and produced the fewest actual changes in the practice of standard obstetrics. Although the wholesale outlawing of alternative practices by official medicine risked alienating their clientele, the creation of visual alterations to their practice of birth made professional medicine appear conciliatory to consumer demands, while maintaining medical control and authority over birth. The alternative birth centers and labor-delivery-recovery rooms in these hospitals were more of a hook for clients than actual alternative locations. For example, one attending physician stated, "I have control all the time. . . . Only because I feel that I am very much in control in the ABC [alternative birth center] am I able to relinquish some of that control to [my patients]. . . . I'm running the show—in the ABC more than anywhere else. You have more of a feeling that you have control, and on most of my patients, in fact, I would say all of them, I have absolute control over them. . . . I permit them the opportunity to run the show . . . but they understand that I'm in there and I'm the boss." Although hospital-based birth centers suggested a compromise by professional medicine and many women have had productive, positive birth experiences in these, often in these centers there has been no real attempt to limit technical or medical interventions—protocol remained unaltered. For example, time limits were imposed on labor. If a woman did not progress according to these standards, complications were "identified" and invasive steps were taken, ranging from the induction of labor to transfer to a standard delivery room to a cesarean section. As Dr. Martha Illige-Saucier, a Denver obstetrician, stated, "My concern is that [these centers] are a case of the emperor's new clothes, where there's a lot of trumpeting and thundering, but things aren't any different than they have been." These programs in "interior decorating obstetrics," as Dr. Barbara Katz Rothman calls them, attracted patients and cut costs while paying lip-service to the idea of birth as normal.[62] However, few women actually experienced such a birth. These alternative birth centers were, in effect, a move toward consolidation of authority to the medical profession.

A renewed interest in birth chairs further illustrated this trend toward "compromise" with a more natural perception of birth and the subtle and not-so-subtle efforts toward a consolidated practice of medicalized birth. Starting in the mid-1970s, advertisements began to appear in mainstream obstetrical journals for devices such as birth chairs and labor-delivery-recovery beds, often referred to as "chair-beds." Although the first companies to advertise in journals were alternative ones such as the Family Birth Center and Obstetrics Diversified, by 1979 medical manufacturing companies like Century Manufacturing, the Borning Corporation (now a subsidiary of Hill-Rom, Inc.), and Stryker Medical (formerly Stryker/Adel Manufacturing) were also advertising birth chairs and chair-beds for use in hospital settings in publications such as *The Journal of the American Medical Association, American Journal of Obstetrics and Gynecology,* and *Obstetrics and Gynecology.* This reintroduction of birth chairs and the introduction of chair-beds in the late 1970s and 1980s by medical manufacturing companies was an effort to appear in step with the trend of alternative birth, while profiting from and controlling the movement.

The promotional materials for these items clearly convey the idea of compromise. For example, Century Manufacturing advertised their birth chair as "a more natural and comfortable position; returning back to basics."[63] A Borning Corporation advertisement stated the following about their beds, "Once, care could be responsive to the family's emotional needs during the most significant event of their lives. . . . Or it could have the safety of uncompromised standard medical care. Now it can be both."[64] However, the marketing material for these items also dwelled on their many medical and operative attributes, thus reassuring hospitals and doctors of little alteration or interference in the conventional process.[65]

An example is the "Century Birthing Chair," which is a fiberglass mold-

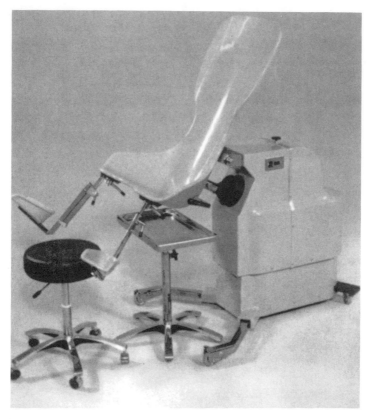

Figure 3.10. The "Century Birthing Chair," American, c. 1980s.
Manufactured and marketed by Century Manufacturing Company.
Photograph courtesy of Century Manufacturing Company.

ed chair with stainless steel footrests, hand-holds attached to the seat, an adjustable tray stand for tools and equipment, and a hydraulic lift that can be raised and lowered (Figure 3.10). The seat height varies from approximately twenty-two inches to more than thirty inches, and the seat opening is eight inches across. The entire chair can be situated in any number of vertical or horizontal angles, all controlled by a doctor-operated foot pedal.[66]

The Century chair was a compromise—suggesting alternative birth, but incorporating all the perceived elements of the medical approach. It also had many aspects that were not conducive and acceptable to the woman delivering. Once in the chair, it was difficult for the woman to get out of it, which curtailed her freedom of movement during labor. With poor foot support for bracing, the position of the woman's body placed additional pressure to her bottom, which, according to women's complaints, increased the incidence of painful back labor and hemorrhoids. Because the doctor controlled the foot pedals, once the mother was in the chair she had little say over the position she was placed in and little freedom to control the process.[67]

However, complaints about the Century chair did not only come from women. In fact, even with the medical elaborations, complaints were much more vehement among medical personnel using these items. Although the major manufacturers of contemporary birth chairs sought to minimize these complaints, doctors argued that the new birth chairs did not have the options of different positions and the chairs impeded operative deliveries. When questioned about birth chairs, many doctors dismissed them as a passing fad. Doctors' remarks such as, "I don't like them," "Chairs are inconvenient," or "Well, they are one of those cute things," make it apparent that the reappearance of birth chairs in professional obstetrics was not based on any fundamental change in the philosophy of birth, but was rather a reaction to underlying economic issues.[68] The continued complaints from doctors, the limited use, and quick dismissal of birth chairs reveal that their reappearance was only a gesture at compromise.[69]

Birth chairs like the Century chair, not to mention the more alternative designs, never found widespread use with professional obstetricians in the United States because their use would have required an alteration to the very basic philosophy of medicalized birth. While St. Joseph's Hospital in Wichita, Kansas, offered a birth chair in 1979, this option was no longer offered in 1986 because the "fad" had died out.[70] Birth-chair manufacturers, such as Century Manufacturing and Affiliated Hospital Products, discontinued production of birth chairs in the late 1980s and early 1990s due to low sales.[71] Hospitals discovered they could attract business and appear to be compromising through their alternative birth centers, labor-delivery-recovery rooms, and the new obstetrics "chair-beds" without the great concession of providing birth chairs. By the mid-1980s, offering birth chairs in hospitals as a response to demands of society and the consumer market had run its course. Birth chairs were thrown away, put into storage, or shipped to disadvantaged hospitals in foreign countries as tax deductions.[72]

However, labor-delivery-recovery beds, or chair-beds, designed by medical manufacturing companies became quite popular. These new designs,

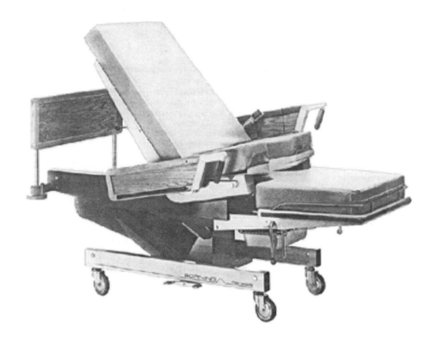

Figure 3.11. Birthing bed, American, c. 1980s. Manufactured by the Borning Corporation. Reproduction taken from publicity materials courtesy of the Borning Corporation.

which were similar to standard hospital beds, were used in the labor-delivery-recovery rooms. These beds provided hospitals with something to indicate that they were receptive to the "natural experience" and still on the cutting edge of birth technology, but actually altered hospitals' chosen and understood approach to delivery very little. Labor-delivery-recovery beds were basically standard hospital beds with a group of moveable sections that could accommodate any position from semiupright birth to complete horizontal delivery with stirrups and restraints. The beds featured a pull-away lower section that created a narrow ledge, like a seat, in the middle. These beds offered the option of upright delivery, like that in a birth chair. They could also be lowered for operative deliveries, be positioned for lithotomy

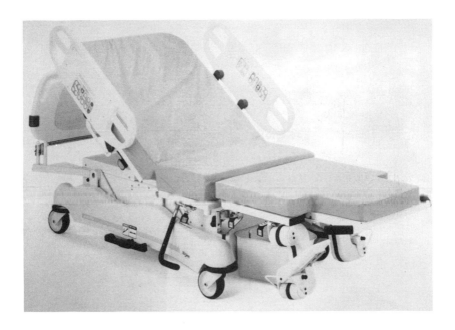

Figure 3.12. The "First Care Ultra" delivery bed, American, 1998. Manufactured by Stryker Medical, Kalamazoo, Michigan. Photograph courtesy of Stryker Medical.

birth, serve as a postpartum or recovery bed, and be used to roll the woman down the hall to an operating room should complications require.

As a testament to the intent of their manufacturers to be innovative and responsive, these beds passed through numerous designs. All had braces, hand-holds, and squatting bars. Some beds, such as the later ones designed by Borning, even featured a wedge opening shaped by the mattress when the lower portion was pulled away (Figure 3.11). Stryker Medical's "Stretcher Bed" and, more recently, the "First Care Ultra" offered many of the same elements on their beds. Stryker advertised the option of at least nine different positions for labor, birth, and recovery, and additional features that made even operative delivery possible.[73] The latest design from Stryker Medical now also features an optional "V-cut" seat as well (Figure 3.12).

Borning's latest design, the "Affinity II Birthing Bed," is advertised with the following options: hinged foot section, pelvis tilt, instrument and CPR attachment, calf supports, side rails, and seat shapes in both the wedge and straight-edge options. Such innovations reveal the prevailing philosophy behind this artifact. Regardless of the innovations in design, with so many options and fall-backs, the company was clearly interpreting birth as a medical event.

Unlike the new designs of birth chairs, labor-delivery-recovery beds were popular with doctors because, while offering alternative postures, they required or demanded no real alteration to the basic medical philosophy and approach to birth. These beds were also more cost efficient because they were used for all stages of the woman's hospital stay. Although all designs of birthing beds allowed more options in posture, they were clearly items of medicine, featuring and advertised as having all the "necessary" elements for a medical birth. In fact, interviews with student nurse-midwives reveal that often the very elements that made these labor-delivery-recovery beds useful to women in upright delivery, principally the bracing bar attachment that fit over the wedge seat, were missing and had to be hunted down in distant hospital storage rooms. This could certainly be interpreted as a means to control birth by "hiding" away the innovative article that could alter the posture and, thus, possibly the perception of the birth act.[74]

Consolidation and Repudiation

Simultaneous with such visual compromises in labor-delivery-recovery rooms and birthing centers, the artifacts of hospital birth make clear that professional medicine was also attempting to consolidate control. As professional obstetrics had done in the nineteenth century, modern professional medicine responded to what they perceived as threats to their professional authority by creating and implementing highly elaborate and interventionist procedures. Professional medicine used its advanced technology to argue both for medical intervention and against natural birth. Some examples of these new techniques are amniocentesis, chorionic villus sampling, ultrasound, fetal monitoring strips, maternal blood tests, alpha-fetoprotein, embryoscopy, and the Fetal Pelvic Index (a formula that can "identify" those women who should attempt vaginal delivery and those who should automatically schedule a cesarean section).[75]

Advocacy for medical intervention, both in tests and practices, is evidence of the success of the effort to control the medical understanding and approach to birth. This is also evident in the marked increase in cesarean-section rates that paralleled the growth of the alternative birth movement.[76] In sharp contrast to European cesarean-section rates, in the United States cesarean-section rates were 4.0 percent in 1965, 10.4 percent in 1975, 16.5 percent in 1980, and 23.5 percent in 1990.[77] This rate is nearly two to three times that of European countries, including countries with some of the lowest perinatal mortality rates in the world. Significantly, the World Health Organization believes there is no justification for a cesarean-section rate over 10–15 percent.[78] Motivation for such increases is that cesarean sections require the most management by the doctor and the least labor by the woman and have the highest monetary reward.[79] Also, a groundless idea has been proposed that perfect babies result from such nontraumatic births.[80]

As professional obstetrics had done in the nineteenth century, modern professional medicine also responded to what it perceived as threats to professional authority by the systematic repudiation of rivals and the ridiculing of alternative practices. By lobbying local governments and state medical boards; instituting rigorous licensing, state inspections, and regulations; establishing insurance requirements for any free-standing birth centers; and by vocally and professionally discouraging the use of alternative birth centers, midwives, and nurse-midwives as less than safe attendants, professional medicine moved to reaffirm its philosophy and, therefore, practice of birth.[81] Official medicine dictated what practices were to be considered normative and what atmosphere was to be considered an acceptable one.

In addition, physicians regulated the practice of birth by developing a system of punishment for failing to adhere to the tenets of the group. Through professional ostracism and the discontinuation of malpractice insurance and hospital-admitting privileges, professional organizations often kept midwives and unorthodox physicians from assisting in alternative birth settings. During the nineteenth century, a woman calling in a doctor for a delivery was charged extra if a midwife had been called in first. In the twentieth century, one physician who supported a group of certified nurse-midwives was forced to leave town due to the cancellation of his malpractice insurance and lack of referrals from his "colleagues."[82] These are only two examples of how professional medicine marginalized and even criminalized those who did not cooperate with its standards of behavior and defer to its authority.

At the same time, however, professional medicine encouraged the use of midwives at hospitals where the majority of deliveries were by indigent women, such as General Hospital in Nashville, and in rural areas, such as in Appalachia, where doctors had no interest in practicing. As the head of obstetrics at Vanderbilt Medical Center stated:

I'm impressed that midwives have a place in medicine, but it is not necessarily the place that they [have] always wanted to be. We had some midwives here in town who wanted to have a private practice and compete with the doctors, and that raises some problems. You know you have to have a structure really set up for them and in this town we just didn't need it. There is a place for these people, but I'm just saying that if I had to pick a place, my number one place would be areas where there is an insufficient number of physicians delivering babies. That's where they belong.[83]

In addition to the repudiation of their rivals, obstetricians also publicly campaigned against forms of natural, nonmedical childbirth, making statements such as, "Natural childbirth is for women in rice paddies," and "An infant's safety should take precedence over its mother's emotional needs."[84] Those who chose alternative birth were characterized as "part of a growing rebellion by patients who *challenge* the *judgment* of medical *experts* and question their profits" (emphases added).[85] In the words of a past-president of the Massachusetts Section of the American College of Obstetrics and Gynecology, parents choosing home birth were "kooks, the lunatic fringe, people who have emotional problems that they are acting out."[86] One obstetrician writing in "The Medical Case against Natural Childbirth" even referred to natural childbirth's "un-American" origin as a threat to democracy and womankind.[87] To bolster their opposition, obstetricians wrote articles for women's magazines explaining and rationalizing practices such as routine episiotomies, the use of forceps, and sedation. These patronizing articles, the pressure and often coercive behavior of a woman's personal physician, and the condemnation by official organizations created a formidable barrier for the development of a context for a change in the societal understanding and, therefore, cultural construction of birth.[88] The majority of society was reinforced in the belief that, as Dr. Jerald Coreton stated in 1986, "Pregnancy is an accident going somewhere to happen."[89]

That birth chairs experienced a limited revival in professional obstetrics in the late 1970s and early 1980s, medical manufacturers advertised birth chairs in major obstetrical journals, and a number of standard hospitals created alternative birthing areas all seem to indicate that the alternative birth movement had a considerable effect on the philosophy and practices of both professional medicine and the population it tended. Actually, the history of the birth chair and other artifacts of birth tells a different story.

While the alternative birth movement attempted to reinterpret and redefine the philosophy of birth and thereby secure an accompanying natural approach to delivery, the medical philosophy of birth in the late twentieth century exhibited greater impact on the practice of birth than it ever had before. In-hospital birth chairs and birthing suites and hospital-based midwives appeared not because of any shift in the medical philosophy of birth, but rather because of professional medicine's attempts to maintain control of and access to the highly lucrative field of obstetrics. Although it presented a contest, the alternative movement was unable to produce a context in which professional obstetrics would willingly alter its approach to birth. What the contesting philosophy produced instead was the alteration of certain visual aspects of professional obstetrics. Essentially, it brought about a "face-lift" for delivery. The medical ideology and definition of birth that drove practice remained prevalent in contemporary obstetrics, as seen in the 1978 edition of *The Textbook of Obstetrics and Gynecology:* "Use of the lithotomy position has two purposes: it makes maintenance of asepsis easier and it contributes greatly to the convenience of the obstetrician. These advantages more than compensate for the somewhat unphysiologic posture and the discomfort of the posture itself."[90]

When a show of compromise was necessary to maintain control, professional medicine marketed and occasionally used birth chairs, advocated and introduced more user-friendly climates for birth, and allowed women a modicum of choice in the event. However, the brief presence and occasional use of birth chairs and other devices in standard practice obstetrics were merely a symbol of the alternative, a gesture toward a compromise, not a step away from convention. Acceptance of any practice that allowed consistent and continued use of alternative approaches, such as the use of a birth chair, would have been inconsistent with the driving philosophy. The alternative movement has been thus far unable to create a climate that would radically alter the prevailing philosophy of birth in the way that medicine was able to in the nineteenth century. Without overwhelming motivation for change, the philosophy and the practices remained unaltered. The ultimate triumph of the professional medical philosophy of birth, as seen in the failure of the revival of birth chairs and in the popularity of labor-delivery-recovery beds as artifacts of a medical locale illustrates that the attitudes of professional medicine toward the disease state of pregnancy and birth have not altered. This contest for control of birth and the existence of two vastly different philosophies of birth in the United States reveals clearly how important societal forces are in defining birth. In turn, the way in which these different philosophies have been interpreted and acted upon, as viewed through their associated artifacts, highlights their influential role in shaping the actual practice of delivery.

Notes

1. Leavitt (1984: 176).
2. Gellhorn (1926: 301–302).
3. Hoffert (1989: 71).
4. Mcvoy (1938), quoted in Leavitt (1984: 326).
5. Leavitt (1984).
6. Ehrenreich and English (1973: 34), Stewart (1981: 8). For more information about the demise of midwives and the issues of gender and professionalism in the early twentieth century in the United States, see Borst (1995: 152–160).
7. Finney (1937: 6–7).
8. Hufford (1988: 228).
9. W. Tyler Smith (1847: 458–460).
10. The discussion of the demise of midwives and the medicalization of birth has been treated in much more detail elsewhere. See works such as Arms (1975, 1994); Romalis and Jordan (1981); Oakley (1984); Ashford (1988); Donnison (1988); Davis-Floyd (1992); Davis-Floyd and Sargent (1997); Rooks (1997).
11. J. W. White (1931: 564–572), Wadsworth (1910), Buck (1920).
12. Although Thompson's work on birth chairs can be found only in a few published articles and the reproduction birth chair now in the collection of the London Museum of Science and Industry, the remnants of labels found on a few chairs suggests that he organized an exhibition of the birth chairs then in the collection of the Wellcome Medical History Museum. According to the archive of the Wellcome Institute, it is believed that many of Dr. Thompson's papers were lost during the Second World War.
13. Markoe (1915: 95–101). The chair designed and constructed by Markoe at the Lying-In Hospital in New York City is illustrated in this article.
14. See Jo Oppenheimer (1990). See also Ehrenreich and English (1978).
15. For more information, see Arnup et al. (1990).
16. Howard (1959: 1141).

17. Howard (1959: 1143).

18. Shultz (May 1958: 35–39).

19. Shultz (August 1958: 59).

20. See Martin (1987), Osherson and Singhorn (1981: 218–249).

21. Kosmark (1938), Devitt (1977: 37). A 1983 report on births from 1915 to 1929 indicates that there was a 40–50 percent increase in the number of infants who died because of injuries sustained in delivery and that half of maternal deaths in this period were attributable to interventions. Cited in Wertz and Wertz (1989: 161).

22. This is important because the women served by such services as Mary Breckenridge's Frontier Nursing Service were below the poverty line, with many more physical challenges to a safe and healthy pregnancy and birth. See Breckenridge (1981). For statistics, see Devitt (1977: 55).

23. Lynn K., interview by author, Bloomington, Indiana, 28 March 1993.

24. Karmel (1965: 32).

25. See for example, Ruzek (1978).

26. Kilchenstein (1980). See also Gaskin (1978).

27. In the United States, due to the presence of a nonsocialized medical system where the rewards for medical care were very great, birth remained a highly lucrative and regimented process. Although the economic rewards for very elaborate birth techniques remain great and the lack of governmental or private-sector control provides little or no form of restraint and control for doctors, the development of various managed-care programs have effectively curtailed some highly interventionist techniques, but only to a limited degree. Managed care has stabilized health-care costs; however, it is met with high levels of disapproval among medical professionals and is being presented to the public as unacceptable and mercenary. For example, an episode of the hugely popular television show, "ER" (16 May 1996), focuses on the mercenary, unhelpful, and often cruel quality of managed care. See Klapper (1973: 586–587). See also Towler and Bramall (1986: 288–302), Donnison (1988).

28. As stated earlier, there have been a number of significant social histories of birth that address this transition as well as the development of the crusade for change as embodied in the alternative birth movement. For example, see Romalis and Jordan (1981); Oakley (1984); Wertz and Wertz (1989); Davis-Floyd (1992); Davis-Floyd and Sargent (1997); Rooks (1997). The artifactual approach presented here offers a different way to track these changes and to interpret the societal context that acted as a catalyst.

29. Jones (1991: 2).

30. Hufford (1988: 245–247).

31. Sullivan and Weitz (1988).

32. Ruth Lubic, director of the Maternity Center of New York, interview by author, New York, New York, 11 July 1992.

33. A number have subsequently closed due to liability insurance and licensing problems. Rooks et al. (1989: 1804). See also Eakins (1984: 49–64).

34. Statistics courtesy of the American College of Nurse-Midwives, telephone

conversations with author, 15 May 1992 and the National Center of Health Statistics at the Center for Disease Control in Atlanta, http://www.cdc.gov/nchs/. See also Rooks (1997).

35. Fitzgerald (1990: A1).

36. In its first five years, ninety-two percent of the 2,050 patients at the Childbearing Center of Douglas General Hospital in Georgia received no painkillers. Mortality was 12.2 per 1,000 births in 1980, the center's first year, but it dropped to 2.2 per 1,000 births the following year. This is compared to the national average at the time of 12.5 infant deaths per 1,000 births. Greene (1983: 36).

37. Marsden G. Wagner, "Infant Mortality in Europe: Implications for the United States," *Journal of Public Health Policy* (Winter 1988), quoted in Jones (1991: 3). Billiter (1992), Trunzo (1989).

38. Friedland (1986).

39. Romond and Baker (1985).

40. See the *Birth and Family Journal* 4 (1977): 79.

41. Personal correspondence, Valerie Appleton, Moonflower Birthing Supply, 16 February 1993.

42. Ruth Lubic, Maternity Center of New York, interview by author, New York, New York, 11 July 1992.

43. Lessa Ginther, Woman Care, Inc., letter to author, 29 June 1992. Ruth Lubic, Maternity Center of New York, interview by author, New York, New York, 11 July 1992. Sharon P., interviews by author, Philadelphia, Pennsylvania, 6 April 1992 and 27 July 1992. Lenora K., interview by author, Washington, D.C., 25 October 1992.

44. Personal correspondence, Lessa Ginther, Woman Care, Inc., letter to author, 29 June 1992.

45. Richard Jennings, director of The Birthing Suite, Pennsylvania Hospital, interview by author, Philadelphia, Pennsylvania, 13 July 1992.

46. Richard Jennings, director of The Birthing Suite, Pennsylvania Hospital, interview by author, Philadelphia, Pennsylvania, 13 July 1992.

47. Advertisement in *Journal of Nurse-Midwifery* (1979: vol. 24).

48. Krepple (1984). See also Hosford (1976), Goldstein (1983), McDowell (1984).

49. Leavitt (1984: 5) provides a graph that charts the number of articles on women's health. For examples, see McCormack (1981), Cates (1982), Rutenberg (1983), Elias (1986), Kotulak (1987). For examples of dissertations and theses on this topic, see Wheeler (1979), Lubic (1980), McSwain (1980).

50. Melanie L., letters to author, 14 November 1992, 26 January 1993.

51. The birth rate in 1959 was 25.7 births per 1,000 people, reached a low in 1973 with 14.5 births per 1,000 and increased to 16.5 births per 1,000 in 1983. This increase in the 1980's was due to the baby boomers reaching the prime childbearing ages of 25–34. See Goodman (1985).

52. Lerman (1991).

53. Chris Clark, R.N., Baptist Hospital, interview by author, Nashville, Tennessee, 29 July 1992. Dr. Richard Jennings, director of The Birthing Suite, Pennsylvania Hospital, interview by author, Philadelphia, Pennsylvania, 13 July 1992.

54. The Baptist Hospital of Nashville hosted a "Childbirth Fair" in April 1992 with classes in breast feeding, early pregnancy, creative solutions to child care, and preparing baby's nursery. Swingley (1992).

55. Vinay (1985: 23).

56. Parachini (1987).

57. Parachini (1987: 1).

58. Channing (1848: 223).

59. DeVries (1983: 7).

60. For example, in 1991 the monthly transfer rate of the Birthing Suite of Pennsylvania Hospital ranged between 20 and 29 percent. Dr. Richard Jennings, director of The Birthing Suite, Pennsylvania Hospital, interview by author, Philadelphia, Pennsylvania, 13 July 1992. The transfer rate of women out of alternative birth areas during labor to standard delivery rooms in the early 1980s was very high, averaging 22.58 percent. DeVries (1983: 6).

61. Vinay (1985: 12).

62. Rothman (1983: 5).

63. Century Manufacturing Company, letter to author, 19 March 1990.

64. Advertisement in the *American Journal of Obstetrics and Gynecology* 143 (1980). A Century birth chair cost $5,000 in January 1981 and $5,400 by October 1981.

65. For example, the marketing materials for the Borning 650 H-R Birth Chair/Childbearing Bed and the Borning Genesis Birthing-Bed. Publicity materials courtesy of Jean Bergwell, The Borning Corporation, Spokane, Washington (now Hill-Rom, Inc., a subsidiary of Hillenbrand, Battesville, Indiana).

66. Promotional and advertising materials, Century Manufacturing Company, 1990.

67. For example, Goodlin (1983: 334).

68. Toni J., Margaret W., and Hillary S.; interviews by author; Philadelphia, Pennsylvania; 17 July 1992 and 6 August 1992.

69. In many European countries where midwife attendance is the norm and some alternative forms of birth are practiced, birth chairs are accepted as a real alternative to the standard recumbent birth postures. For example, Dr. Ingvar Haukeland (1981: 116) stated that birth chairs in Norway "satisfy the requirements of present-day obstetrics." For examples of European attitudes toward birth chairs, see Geiger (1966), Méndez-Bauer et al. (1975), Schurz (1981), Kesby (1982), Nagai (1982), Valenti et al. (1982), Stewart et al. (1983), Berg and Selbing (1984), Liddell et al. (1985).

70. Mines (1988: 13).

71. Century Manufacturing Company, telephone conversation with author, 8 February 1993.

72. McKibben (1989: 47).

73. Jean Bergwell, The Borning Corporation, a subsidiary of Hill/Rom, Inc.,

telephone conversation with author, 25 January 1994. Stryker Adel Corporation, letter to author, 2 February 1994.

74. Personal communication, Robbie Davis-Floyd, 5 January 1999.

75. Rothman (1993).

76. High cesarean rats are only one reflection of the unnecessary and expensive medical procedures that became very common for women. Recent studies have shown that in most cases of breast cancer, less radical lumpectomy followed by radiation therapy was just as effective as a mastectomy. However, nine of ten women diagnosed with breast cancer still have mastectomies. Likewise, a study by the Rand Corporation of 642 hysterectomies found that only fifty-eight percent could be termed "medically appropriate." See *Glamour* (September 1993: 129). See also Anders (1993) and "Study Supports Suspicions About C-Sections, Researchers Say," *The Washington Post*, 20 January 1993.

77. Statistics courtesy of the American College of Obstetricians and Gynecologist, telephone conversation with author, 4 January 1993.

78. World Health Organization (1985: 432). See also Jones (1991: 13). The cesarean-section rates, extensive prenatal testing and treatment, and medication are all examples of the power and preeminence of the medical philosophy of birth, which is in direct contradiction of study after study indicating that such heroic measures are not only unnecessary, but excessive and dangerous. U.S. Preventative Services Task Force (1993).

79. Metropolitan Life Insurance Company listed the average cost for a cesarean section in 1990 as $8,530, with the mid-Atlantic states of New Jersey, New York, and Pennsylvania having the highest number performed (34.3 percent). In comparison, a vaginal delivery costs an average of $1,800. In Metropolitan Life managed-care programs, all deliveries are scheduled for a flat fee, vaginal and cesarean deliveries costing the same, whereas their standard health insurance policies pay rates based on procedures performed. Metropolitan Life reports that women in the managed care programs have a distinctly lower cesarean-section rate than their individual standard policy holders. "Charges for a Cesarean Section: United States, 1990," *MET Statistical Bulletin* 73 (January/March 1992): 12–18. Carrie B., conversation with author, Nashville, Tennessee, 23 April 1993.

80. A study by Cleveland doctor Frederick J. Roemer reported that children delivered by scheduled cesarean sections and who experienced no labor had I.Q.s ten points higher than their siblings who had unscheduled cesarean sections and experienced some labor. Although the study had many sampling problems and any real conclusive evidence is unattainable, this study was widely publicized. Vrazo (1991).

81. In fact, numerous studies reveal that nurse-midwives, midwives, birth centers, and other alternative birth practices have a very high success rate for both mother and child. Although critics argue that those choosing alternative forms of delivery are self-selective (in that those prone to high-risk births rarely choose such approaches and that this affects the percentage of success), such characterization fails to

account for the overall positive percentages. For a number of these studies, see Rooks (1997). See also MacDorman and Singh (1998).

82. Rosen (1946: 123). Many insurance companies will not cover a delivery outside a standard and accepted hospital or clinic, regardless of the safety and licenses held by the alternative establishment.

83. Dr. Frank Boehm, interview by author, Nashville, Tennessee, 6 August 1992.

84. *Newsweek* (1965: 98), Friedland (1986: 1).

85. Cates (1982: 1).

86. DeVries (1983: 4).

87. Fielding and Benjamin, *The Childbirth Challenge* (1962); Fielding and Benjamin *McCall's* (1962: 106–107).

88. For example, see Gerbie (1967).

89. de Kruif (1936), Friedland (1986: 1).

90. Quoted in Simon (1983: 175).

Belief, Artifacts, and the Cultural Construction of Medicine

From the sixteenth to the late twentieth century, the practice of birth changed radically. The history of birth within a biosocial framework, one that "is produced jointly and reflexively by (universal) biology and (particular) society" helps us to understand why these changes took place and how the many elements involved.[1] Artifacts of birth allow us to mark the progress of changes in practice as well as identify the attendant rationale and beliefs that are influencing these practices—the philosophy of birth. The cultural construction of birth that is thus revealed incorporates the philosophy of birth and the associated practices of delivery.

During this period, societal forces culminated to provide the impetus, resources, and context for a drastic reinterpretation of the philosophy of birth. Such a redefinition was made manifest in the artifacts of birth. The changes in the practice and the artifacts of birth are evidence of the rise of the medical profession with its attendant academic surroundings, technical practices, economic power, and prevailing philosophy. The increasing pre-eminence of the physician drove the changes in the practice of birth and spelled doom for the traditional practice of midwifery. This increased involvement of doctors altered the philosophy of birth by systematically redefining pregnancy and birth as pathology that required medical treatment and encouraging childbearing women to view their condition as one demanding medical care and cure that only male medical professionals could adequately provide. This redefinition of birth advocated an increasingly interventionist approach, thus altering the practice and the cultural construction of birth.

The development of the professional medical philosophy of birth continued until the middle years of this century, when a movement for alternative birth began to challenge it. Women began to question some of the procedures shaped by professional obstetrics and, by extension, the prevailing medical philosophy. Diametrically opposed philosophies of birth that were motivated and shaped by different societal issues now operated within society. The appearance of an alternative, or revived, natural philosophy of birth was stimulated by a variety of reasons, but primarily by the renewed contact and community of women, the development of a self-help movement in society, and legitimate publicized concerns about the treatment of birth. The alternative birth movement presented a philosophy of birth as natural and nonmedical and proposed practices based on the reality of the event rather than ideological and technical issues. This movement for change and the accompanying reappraisal of the prevailing medical philosophy of birth infiltrated, to a limited extent, the standard professional obstetrical approach to delivery. Physicians accepted some alterations to the practice of delivery, although the alternative birth movement did not bring about a real shift in the prevailing philosophy of birth. The medical profession eventually responded with a movement toward greater consolidation and the creation and implementation of tests and procedures that further controlled the process of birth as a medical event.[2]

However, this history of birth, particularly of the contemporary struggle for authority to define belief and dictate practice, plays only one part in the larger history of the competition between official medicine and community-based or alternative medicine.[3] The response of medical professionals to the challenges to their authority to dictate practices reveals that birth was only one small aspect of a systematic redefinition of human conditions as medical events, which was intended to bolster the authority that society cedes to physicians. The durability of the medical philosophy of birth illustrates the readiness of the general public to accept the authority of science and portrays a general societal deference to professionalism in idea and in practice. This deference represents a long-term shift in the entire cultural construction of care and practice and of the growth in scientific authority.

The similarities between the shift toward medical intervention in birth and the shift in the general philosophy of health care provokes unavoidable comparisons. The shift toward the authority of medicine and science is evident in the artifacts of medicine, daily life, and culture. Studying the philosophy and associated practice provides a way to highlight the important influences and effects of changing social attitudes about on other areas of health.

Such a comparison suggests changes in attitudes toward childbearing and women, as well as a radical change in the social definition and interpretation of disease; the qualifications for and the authority of health-care providers; and a willingness to rely, without question, on specialists for care and cure. As in the birth process, professional medicine has shaped social beliefs and influenced cultural practices for the life cycle by creating and cultivating medical definitions for the critical junctures. There are many examples in typical health care provided to women from birth through middle age, including medical exams at menarche, blood tests and genetic counseling at marriage, medical tests and treatment during pregnancy, hospital delivery, high rates of cesarean delivery, and estrogen therapy at menopause.

By the introduction of many aspects of care and treatment that coincide and mark these various stages, doctors and professional medicine have taught society what to think and how to behave. For example, hyperactivity and depression have been treated as a chemical imbalances and social concerns such as smoking, alcoholism, and criminality have been alleged to be chemical or physical manifestations in the brain.[4] By naming and treating both environmental and cultural disorders, the profession of medicine, as did the church authorities for hundreds of years before, has cast itself as a social agent. The profession has become intimately involved in the construction and regulation of norms of social behavior, which it justifies by scientific explanations.

The repackaging of traditional health practices and treatments by medical professionals offers vivid examples of the way in which official medicine has created an aura of unquestioned superiority and the authority to dictate and drive practice. The "discovery" of the use of ergot in delivery from a midwife by Dr. John Sterns and Withering's "discovery" of foxglove (digitalis) are classic examples of professional medicine appropriating previously rejected, traditional artifacts and practices and presenting them as medical advances, thus providing scientific rationale and accepting the plaudits for invention.[5]

The ebb and flow of the medical argument first *against* and then *for* breast-feeding infants is another example of the right of professional medicine to dictate behavior and influence practice through artifact analysis. Study of baby bottles and other items of infant feeding, associated advertisements, pertinent articles in women's magazines, and medical literature detail not just the chronological history, but also the shifts in understandings and in attitudes toward breast-feeding.

These items, like birth chairs, reveal that by creating a mentality of deference to medical authority in society, anything associated with medical practice automatically gained acceptance, whether it was useful, original, or not. However, we are taught by the medical profession to question all "nonscientific" things. Society only gives widespread acceptance to devices and practices when they are driven by medical ideology and sanctioned by medical practice. The medical philosophy clearly shaped and molded society's beliefs in accordance with its prevailing ideology, shaped and drove the associated practices, and therefore shaped and influenced the cultural construction of contemporary medical care.

This ascendancy of professional medicine as an agent of social control further strengthens the premise that the prevailing medical philosophy shapes attitude and practice, where form drives function.[6] Differences in opinion are quickly labeled deviant and adherents are marginalized. This is apparent in the efforts of professional medicine to marginalize practitioners of alternative birth as well as the continued struggle with chiropractors, the vitamin and herbal-remedy industry, and other self-help movements and, particularly, in the social, political, legal, and medical responses to fundamental Christian healing beliefs.[7] Women who refused cesarean sections or practiced unaccepted approaches to birth were once charged with witchcraft. Now they are subject to lawsuits. Also, parents are charged with neglect if they withhold medical care from their children due to ideology or religious belief.

As society moves toward a total reliance on medical interpretations, it also embraces science and technology. Doctors and scientists have advocated and detailed means for scientific housekeeping, scientific childrearing, and scientific models of education. This growth in social deference to scientific authority and reason has encouraged further reliance on scientific medicine, where doctors prescribed what society does and does not do, thus effectively influencing society in its practices and beliefs.[8]

The two strikingly different histories of birth chairs and birth practices by Savonarola and Dempsey presented at the beginning of this book revealed different philosophies of birth as well. The study of the birth chair, specifically, and of artifacts of birth, in general, further illustrates the significance of these historical differences. This material history frames the associated philosophies of birth by systematically presenting the way in which birth chairs and other artifacts of birth were conceived, designed, built, used, reinterpreted, and dismissed. Over time, the shifts in the philosophy of birth reveal that the alterations in practice (in construction and use of birth chairs) reflect more than current knowledge and understandings of the process of birth alone. Varying societal forces (changes in ideas about women, notions of medical professionalism, and other fundamental elements of the cultural context) converge to define the authority of the principal birth practitioners and, by association, the authority to interpret the birth process, define birth, and dictate processes and procedures. Birth chairs reveal patterns of cultural definition as they change in form and function in response to societal influences and alterations in the prevailing philosophy of birth. In conjunction with a study of cultural and societal issues of the time, the history of any artifact can reveal the society's philosophy and its attendant practices, thus encapsulating and visually displaying their cultural construction and its changes over time.

Notes

1. Jordan (1993: 3).

2. This alternative movement is often accused of romanticizing earlier times by ignoring the number of women who died. It is important to remember that the majority of maternal and infant deaths in earlier times was not so much due to the inefficiency of the prevailing birth practices, but to hygiene, unhealthy living conditions, epidemics from bacteria, and, later, corset use and other elements of fashion. This can be supported by the maternal and infant mortality rates in most Third World countries today stemming from such causes as malnutrition, overwork, and anemia. The drop in mortality rates in the twentieth century was not so much due to leaps in technology and the practice of medicalized obstetrics, but improved living conditions, antibiotics, diet, and hygiene. See Goer (1995), Rooks (1997), and Davis-Floyd (1998).

3. For an in-depth discussion of the sovereignty and social transformation of American medicine, see Starr (1982). See also Birenbaum (1981: 67–82).

4. For a discussion of the change in the designation of social concerns and deviance to illness, see Conrad and Schneider (1980).

5. See Hufford (1988: 228–264).

6. Myerhoff and Larsen (1965: 188–193) discuss the role of doctors as "culture heroes."

7. Hufford (1988: 228–264) discusses the modern images of folk medicine and the medical labeling of folk healers as "quacks." See also Kleinman (1980).

8. Ehrenreich and English (1978: ch. 4).

Appendix:
Museums and Archives with Birth Chairs in Their Collections

Austria

Hallstätter Museum
Fredsgatan 2
A-4830 Hällstatt
Austria

Institute für Geschichte der Medizin
der Universität Wien
Währinger Straße 25
A-1090 Vienna
Austria

Oberösterreiches Landesmuseum
Museumstraße 14
A-4010 Linz
Austria

France

Musee Alsacien
Musees de la Ville de Strasbourg
23 Quai Saint-Nicolas
67000 Strasbourg
France

Germany

Deutsches Medizinhistorisches
Museum
Anatomiestraße 18-20
D-8070 Ingolstadt
Germany

Germanisches Nationalmuseum
Postfach 95 80
850 Nürnberg 11
Germany

Institut für Geschichte der Medizin
der Georg-August-Universität
Nikolausbergerweg 7b
3400 Göttingen
Germany

Stadtmuseum Güntersloh
Kökerstraße 7 9
Postfach 2952
4830 Güntersloh
Germany

Switzerland

Medizinhistorisches Institut und
Museum der Universität Zürich
Rämistraße 69/71
CH-8006 Zürich
Switzerland

United Kingdom

The London Hospital Medical
College
University of London
Turner Street
London E1 2AD
England

The National Museum of Science
and Industry
Science Museum of London
Exhibition Road
London SW7 2DD
England

Royal College of Surgeons
Nicholson Street
Edinburgh EH8 9DW
Scotland

United States

The Cupola House
P.O. Box 474
Edenton, North Carolina 27932

The Hemingway Museum
907 Whitehead Street
Key West, Florida 33040

Thomas Jefferson University
Archives
Scott Building, Room 310
1020 Walnut Street
Philadelphia, Pennsylvania 19107

Museum of Pharmacy and Medicine
10910 East Tanque Verde
Tucson, Arizona 85749

The Mütter Museum
The College of Physicians of
Philadelphia
19 South 22nd Street
Philadelphia, Pennsylvania 19104

University of Kansas Medical Center
The Clendening Library
39th and Rainbow Boulevard
Kansas City, Kansas 66103

Waring Historical Library
Medical University of
South Carolina
171 Ashley Avenue
Charleston, South Carolina
29425-3001

Bibliography

Adams, Alice E. *Reproducing the Womb: Images of Childbirth in Science, Feminist Theory, and Literature.* Ithaca, N.Y.: Cornell University Press, 1994.

Adamson, P. B. "Some Rituals Associated with Parturition in Antiquity." *Folklore* 96 (1985): 176–183.

Ames, Kenneth. "Meaning in Artifacts: Hall Furnishings in Victorian America." *Journal of Interdisciplinary History* 9 (1978): 19–46.

Anders, George. "Surge in Caesareans Appears to Be Tied To Doctors' Malpractice Insurance Rates." *The Wall Street Journal,* 20 January 1993, B6.

Arms, Suzanne. *Immaculate Deception: A New Look at Women and Childbirth in America.* Boston: Houghton-Mifflin, 1975.

————. *Immaculate Deception II: Myth, Magic and Birth.* New York: Celestial Arts, 1994.

Arney, William Ray. *Power and the Profession of Obstetrics.* Chicago, Ill.: University of Chicago Press, 1982.

Arnup, Katherine, Andrée Lévesque, and Ruth Roach Pierson, eds. *Delivering Motherhood: Maternal Ideologies and Practices in the 19th and 20th Centuries.* New York: Routledge, 1990.

Arthure, H. "The Midwife—In Simpson's Time and Ours." *Journal of Obstetrics and Gynaecology of the British Commonwealth* 80 (1973): 1–9.

Ashford, Janet Isaacs. *The Whole Birth Catalog: A Sourcebook for Choices in Childbirth.* Trumansburg, N.Y.: Crossing Press, 1983.

————. *George Engelmann and "Primitive" Birth.* Solana Beach, Calif.: Janet Isaacs Ashford, 1988.

————. *Mothers and Midwives: A History of Traditional Childbirth.* Encinitas, Calif.: Janet Isaacs Ashford, 1988.

Atwood, Margaret E. *The Handmaiden's Tale.* New York: Anchor Books, 1998.

Averling, I. H. *The Chamberlains and the Midwifery Forceps.* London, 1882.

Baker-Benfield, G. J. *The Horrors of the Half-Known Life: Male Attitudes toward Women and Sexuality in Nineteenth-Century America.* New York: Harper & Row, 1976.

Ballantyne, J. W. *The Byrth of Mankynd (Its Authors and Editions).* London: Sherratt & Hughes, 1906.

Bancroft-Livingstone, George. "Louise de la Valliére and the Birth of the Man-Midwife." *Journal of Obstetrics and Gynaecology of the British Empire* 63 (1956): 261–267.

Baudelocque, J. *L'art des accouchemens.* Paris: Mequiqnon, 1796.

Bayerland, Ortloff von. *Das Frauenbüchlein und Arzneibuch,* edited by Gustav Klein. München: Kuhn, 1910.

Bennion, Elisabeth. *Antique Medical Instruments.* Berkeley: University of California Press, 1979.

Bentley, Thomas. *The Monument of Matrones.* London: H. Denham, 1582.

Berg, Göran, and Anders Selbing. "Erfarenheter av en ny typ av förlossningsstol vid kvinnokliniken i Linköping." *Läkartidningen* 81 (1984): 115–118.

Bernstein, Anne. "How Children Learn about Sex and Birth." *Psychology Today* 35 (1976): 31–35.

Bewez, F. O. *Moschionis de mulierum passion ibus liber.* Vienna: Apud Rud Graffer et Soc, 1793.

Biggs, C. Lesley. "The Case of the Missing Midwives: A History of Midwifery in Ontario from 1795 to 1900." In *Delivering Motherhood: Maternal Ideologies and Practices in the 19th and 20th Centuries,* edited by Katherine Arnup, Andrée Lévesque, and Ruth Roach Pierson, 20–35. New York: Routledge, 1990.

Billiter, Bill. "State Regulations, Inspections Urged for Centers to Ensure Quality." *Los Angeles Times,* 6 January 1992, B1, B12.

Birenbaum, Arnold. *Health Care and Society.* Montclair, N.J.: Allanheld, Osmun, 1981.

Bivins, John, Jr., and Paula Welshimer. *Moravian Decorative Arts in North Carolina: An Introduction to the Old Salem Collection.* Salem, N.C.: Old Salem, Inc., 1981.

Black, Matthew, and H. H. Rowley, eds. *Peake's Commentary on the Bible.* Nashville, Tenn.: Thomas Nelson Publishers, 1962.

Blackwell, Elizabeth. *Pioneer Work in Opening the Medical Profession to Women.* New York: Longmans, Green, and Co., 1895.

Boer, Lukas Johann. *Abhandlungen und Versuche zur Begrundung eine neuen, einfachen und naturgemassen Geburtshulfe, und Behandlung der Schwangern, Wochnerinnen, und neugebornen Kinder, sowohl im gesunden als kranken Zustande.* Vienna: Johann George Ritter von Mosle, 1810.

Bogdan, Janet. "Care or Cure? Childbirth Practices in Nineteenth-Century America." *Feminist Studies* 4 (1978): 93–111.

Borst, Charlotte G. *Catching Babies: The Professionalization of Childbirth, 1870–1920.* Cambridge, U.K.: Cambridge University Press, 1995.

Boston Women's Health Book Collective. *The New Our Bodies, Ourselves: A Book by and for Women.* New York: Simon & Schuster, 1984.

Bourgeois, Louise. *The Compleat Midwife's Practice Enlarged in the Most Weighty and High Concernments of the Birth of Man Containing Perfect Directory or Rules for Midwives and Nurses: As Also a Guide for Women in Their Conception, Bearing and Nursing of Children. With Instructions of the Queen of France's Midwife to her Daughter Touching on the Practice of the Said Art.* London: Nathaniel Brook, 1698.

————. *Les Six Couches de Marie de Médicis.* Paris: Leon Willem, 1875.

Brack, D. C. "Displaced: The Midwife by the Male Physicians." *Women and Health* 1 (1976): 18–24.

Bracken, Henry. *The Midwife's Companion; or a Treatise of Midwifery Wherein the Whole Art is Explained.* London: J. Clarke and J. Shuckburgh, 1737.

Breckinridge, Mary. *Wide Neighborhoods: A Story of the Frontier Nursing Service.* Lexington: University Press of Kentucky, 1981.

Briggs, Peter. "Faulty Care and Infant Deaths." *Ladies Home Journal* 62 (September 1955): 122–155.

Bronner, Simon J. "Material Culture." In *An Encyclopedia of American Folklore,* edited by Jan H. Brunvand, 463–466. New York: Garland Publishing, 1996.

Brooks, Juanita. "Frontier Birth Beliefs." *Folklore Forum* 29 (1970): 53–55.

Browne, Alan, ed. *Masters, Midwives and Ladies-in-Waiting: The Rotunda Hospital 1745–1995.* Dublin: The Governors of the Rotunda Hospital, 1995.

Buchanan, William. *Advice to Mothers on the Subject of Their Own Health; and on the Means of Promoting the Health, Strength, and Beauty of Their Off-Spring.* New York: Richard Scott, 1813.

Buck, Albert Henry. *The Dawn of Modern Medicine: An Account of Science and Art of Medicine Which Took Place in Western Europe.* New Haven, Conn.: Yale University Press, 1920.

Bullough, Vern. *The Development of Medicine as a Profession.* New York: S. Karger, 1966.

Burns, John. *The Principles of Midwifery, Including the Diseases of Women and Children.* Philadelphia, Pa.: Hopkins & Earle, 1810.

Carter, Jenny. *With Child: Birth through the Ages.* New York: Mainstream, 1986.

Cassar, P. "Vestiges of the Parturition Chair in Malta." *St. Luke's Hospital Gazette* 8 (1973): 58–60.

Cates, Ellen. "Is It Wrong to Have Babies at Home?" *United Press International,* 4 September 1982, Lifestyles.

Chaney, Judith. "Birthing in Early America." *Journal of Nurse-Midwifery* 25 (1980): 5–13.

Channing, Walter. *A Treatise on Etherization in Childbirth, Illustrated by Five Hundred and Eighty-One Cases.* Boston: W. D. Ticknor and Co., 1848.

Chen, Henry Lin. *Power, Control, and the Right to Birth: The Historical Development of the Obstetrician-Mother Relationship and Its Effect on the Obstetrical Malpractice Crisis.* M.A. thesis, Department of History and Science, Harvard University, 1993.

Cianfrani, Theodore. *A Short History of Obstetrics and Gynecology.* Springfield, Ill.: Charles C. Thomas, 1960.

Conrad, Peter, and Joseph W. Schneider. *Deviance and Medicalization: From Badness to Sickness.* St. Louis, Mo.: C. V. Mosby Company, 1980.

Cooke, Edward S. "The Study of American Furniture from the Perspective of the Maker." In *Perspectives on American Furniture,* edited by Gerald W. R. Ward. New York: W. W. Norton & Co., 1988.

Cope, Zachary, ed. *Sidelights on the History of Medicine.* London: Butterworth and Co. Ltd., 1957.

Cott, Nancy. *A Heritage of Her Own: Toward a New Social History of American Women.* New York: Simon and Schuster, 1969.

————. *Roots of Bitterness: Documents of the Social History of American Women.* New York: Dutton, 1972.

————. *The Bonds of Womanhood: "Women's Sphere" in New England, 1780–1835.* New Haven, Conn.: Yale University Press, 1977.

Cottrell, Barbara. "Effect of the Birth Chair on Duration of Second Stage Labor and Maternal Outcome." *Nursing Research* 35 (1986): 364–367.

Crawford, Patricia M. *Exploring Women's Past: Essays in Social History.* Boston: Allen & Unwin, 1983.

Croutier, Alev Lyte. *Harem: The World behind the Veil.* New York: Abbeville Press, 1989.

Cuisenier, Jean. *French Folk Art.* Tokyo: Kodamoka, 1977.

Culpepper, Nicholas. *A Directory for Midwives; or, a Guide for Women, in Their Conception, Bearing, and Suckling Their Children.* London: J. Streater, 1671.

Curtis, A. *Lectures on Midwifery and the Forms of Disease Peculiar to Women and Children, Delivered to the Members of the Botanico-Medical College of Ohio.* Columbus, Ohio: Jonathan Phillips, 1841.

Daly, Ann. *Inventing Motherhood: The Consequences of an Ideal.* New York: Schocken Books, 1983.

Danforth, David. *The Complete Guide to Pregnancy: An Authoritative Manual for Pregnant Women.* Norwalk, Conn.: Appleton-Century-Crofts, 1984.

Davis-Floyd, Robbie. *Birth as an American Rite of Passage.* Berkeley: University of California Press, 1992.

Davis-Floyd, Robbie, and Carolyn F. Sargent, eds. *Childbirth and Authoritative Knowledge: Cross-Cultural Perspectives.* Berkeley: University of California Press, 1997.

de Kruif, Paul. "Why Should Mothers Die?" *Ladies Home Journal* 53 (1936): 8.

De Lee, J. B. "Meddlesome Midwifery in the Renaissance." *Journal of the American Medical Association* 67 (1916): 1126.

Dempsey, A. J. "A Brief Survey of Early Midwifery Practice." *Ulster Medical Journal* 18 (1949): 109–115.

Deventer, Hendrik van. *Observations Importantes sur le Manuel des Accouchements.* Paris: Pierre-Francois Giffart, 1701.

————. *The Art of Midwifery Improv'd Fully & Plainly Laying down Whatever Instructions Are Requisite to Make a Complete Midwife. And the Many Errors in All the Books Hitherto Written upon This Subject Clearly Refuted.* 3rd ed. London: A. Bettesworth, 1728.

Devitt, Neal. "The Transition from Home to Hospital Birth in the United States, 1930–1960." *Birth and Family Journal* 4 (1977): 47–58.

DeVries, Raymond G. "Image and Reality: An Evaluation of Hospital Alternative Birth Centers." *Journal of Nurse-Midwifery* 28 (1983): 3–9.

————. *Making Midwives Legal: Childbirth, Medicine, and the Law.* Columbus: Ohio State University Press, 1996.

Dickens, Charles. *The Life and Adventures of Martin Chuzzlewit.* New York: Hurts & Co., 1915.

Dietz, Reinboldt. *Sorani Ephesii, De arte obstetricia morbisque mulierium quae supersunt, Regimonti Prussorum.* Köingsberg: Graefium, 1838.

Doble, Gilbert Hunter. *The Saints of Cornwall.* Chatham, U.K.: Parrett & Neves, 1960–1970.

Donegan, Jane B. *Women and Men Midwives: Medicine, Morality, and Misogyny in Early America.* Westport, Conn.: Greenwood Press, 1978.

Donnison, Jean. *Midwives and Medical Men: A History of the Struggle for the Control of Childbirth.* New Barnet, Herts: Historical Publications, Ltd., 1988.

Douglas, Mary. *Purity and Danger: An Analysis of the Concepts of Pollution and Taboo.* London: Ark Paperbacks, 1984.

Drachman, Virginia. "Female Solidarity and Professional Success: The Dilemma of Women Doctors in Late Nineteenth-Century America." *Journal of Social History* 15 (1982): 607–619.

Drinker, Cecil. *Not So Long Ago.* New York: Oxford University Press, 1937.

Duden, Barbara. *The Woman Beneath the Skin: A Doctor's Patients in Eighteenth-Century Germany,* translated by Thomas Dunlop. Cambridge, Mass.: Harvard University Press, 1991.

————. *Disembodying Women: Perspectives on Pregnancy and the Unborn,* translated by Lee Hoinacki. Cambridge, Mass.: Harvard University Press, 1993.

Dye, Nancy Schrom. "History of Childbirth in America." *Signs* 6 (1980): 97–108.

Eakins, Pamela S. "The Rise of the Free Standing Birth Center." *Principles and Practice* 9 (1984): 49–64.

————. *The American Way of Birth.* Philadelphia, Pa.: Temple University Press, 1986.

Ebel, Johann G. *Schilderung des Gebrigsvölkes vom Kanton Glarus.* Leipzig, 1802.

Eberlein, D. E., and Abbot McClure. *The Practical Book of Period Furniture.* Philadelphia, Pa.: J. B. Lippincott & Co., 1914.

Eccles, Audrey. *Obstetrics and Gynaecology in Tudor and Stuart England.* Kent, Ohio: Kent State University Press, 1982.

Edwards, Margot. *Reclaiming Birth: History and Heroines of American Childbirth Reform.* Trumansburg, N.Y.: Crossing Press, 1984.

Edwards, Ralph, ed. *English Chairs.* London: Her Majesty's Stationers Office, 1970.

Edwards, Robert R., and Vickie Ziegler, eds. *Matrons and Marginal Women in Medieval Society.* Woodbridge, Suffolk: Boydell & Brewer, 1995.

Ehrenreich, Barbara. *Witches, Midwives, and Nurses: A History of Women Healers.* Old Westbury, N.Y.: Feminist Press, 1973.

Ehrenreich, Barbara, and Deirdre English. *Complaints and Disorders: The Sexual Politics of Sickness.* Old Westbury, N.Y.: Feminist Press, 1973.

————. *For Her Own Good: 150 Years of the Experts' Advise to Women.* New York: Anchor Books/Doubleday, 1978.

Elias, Marilyn. "Hypnosis for Childbirth Experiencing a Rebirth." *Los Angeles Times,* 8 July 1986, View, Part 5.

Elliger, K., and W. Rudolph, eds. *Biblia Hebraica Stuttgartensia.* Stuttgart: Deutsche Bibelgesellschaft, 1984.

Engelmann, George J. *Labor among Primitive Peoples.* St. Louis, Mo.: J. H. Chambers & Co., 1882.

Erikson, Robert A. *Mother Midnight: Birth, Sex, and Fate in Eighteenth-Century Fiction.* New York: AMS Press, 1986.

Evelyn, D. "Mothers and Their Midwives in Seventeenth-Century London." In *The Art of Midwifery: Early Modern Midwives in Europe,* edited by H. Marland, 9–26. London: Routledge, 1993.

Farber, Gertrude. "Another Old Babylonian Childbirth Incantation." *Journal of Near Eastern Studies* 43 (1984): 311–316.

Fasbender, H. *Geschichte der Geburtshülfe.* Jena, Germany: Fischer, 1906.

Faust, Bernhard Christoph. *Gedanken über Hebammen und Hebammen-anstalten auf dem Lande.* Frankfurt am Main, 1784.

————. *Gütter Rath an frauen über das Gebären.* Hannover, Germany: Gebruder Hahn, 1811.

Feldman, Sylvia. *Choices in Childbirth.* New York: Grosset & Dunlap, 1978.

Fielding, Henry. *Joseph Andrews,* edited by Martin C. Battestin. Boston: Houghton-Mifflin, Riverside Books, 1961.

Fielding, Waldo, and Lois Benjamin. "Medical Case against Natural Childbirth." *McCalls Magazine* 89 (1962): 106–107.

————. *The Childbirth Challenge: Commonsense Versus "Nature" Methods.* New York: Viking Press, 1962.

Findley, Palmer. *Priest of Lucina: The Story of Obstetrics.* Boston: Little, Brown and Co., 1939.

Finney, Roy. *The Story of Motherhood.* New York: Liveright Publishing, 1937.

Fitzgerald, Susan. "Unlicensed But Undaunted: Lay Midwives Seek Legitimacy." *The Philadelphia Inquirer,* 29 April 1990, A1.

Forbes, Thomas Rogers. *The Midwife and the Witch.* New Haven, Conn.: Yale University Press, 1966.

Fox, Claire. "Pregnancy, Childbirth, and Early Infancy in Anglo-American Culture: 1625–1830." Ph.D. diss., Department of American Civilization, University of Pennsylvania, 1966.

Friedenwald, H. "The Physician's Aphorisms: A Medieval Hebrew Satire." *Johns Hopkins Hospital Bulletin* 29 (1918): 69–70.

Friedland, Sandra. "Offering Luxuries Too." *New York Times,* New Jersey edition, 28 September 1986, Section 11, 1.

Gaskin, Ina May. *Spiritual Midwifery.* Summertown, Tenn.: Book Publishing, 1978.

————. "Wanted: Midwives. If We Had More of Them, There Would Be a Lot Less Money Spent on Health Care." *The Tennessean,* 15 November 1993, A10.

Geiger, H. "Über die vertikale Entbindungs methode mittels Gebärstuhl." *Zentralblatt für Gynäkologie* 8 (1966): 229–230.

Gelbart, Nina Rattner. *The King's Midwife: A History and Mystery of Madame du Coundray.* Berkeley: University of California Press, 1998.

Gélis, Jacques. *History of Childbirth,* translated by Rosemary Morris. Boston: Northeastern University Press, 1991.

Gellhorn, G. "New Delivery Bed." *Journal of Obstetrics and Gynecology* 12 (1926): 301–305.

George, Carol, ed. *Remember the Ladies: New Perspectives on Women in America.* Syracuse, N.Y.: Syracuse University Press, 1975.

Gerbie, Albert. "What Happens during Labor?" *Redbook* 129 (1967): 33–34.

Gesenius, Edward. *A Hebrew and English Lexicon of the Old Testament with an Appendix Containing the Biblical Aramaic.* Oxford, U.K.: Clarendon Press, 1951.

Gevitz, Norman. "Three Perspectives on Unorthodox Medicine." In *Other Healers: Unorthodox Medicine in America,* edited by Norman Gevitz, 1–28. Baltimore, Md.: Johns Hopkins University Press, 1988.

Gilman, Charlotte Perkins. *The Yellow Wallpaper.* Old Westbury, N.Y.: The Feminist Press, 1996.

Giron, R. "Attitudes des parturientes." In *Traité de Médicine,* vol. 10, edited by Charles Bouchard, Joseph Babinski, E. Brissaud, and J. M. Charcot. Paris, 1906–1907.

Glassie, Henry. *Pattern in the Material Folk Culture of the Eastern United States.* Philadelphia: University of Pennsylvania Press, 1968.

————. "Meaningful Things and Appropriate Myths: The Artifact's Place in American Studies." In *Material Life in America 1600–1850,* edited by Robert St. George, 63–94. Boston: Northeastern University Press, 1988.

Goer, Henci. *Obstetric Myths Versus Research Realities: A Guide to Medical Literature.* Westport, Conn.: Bergin and Garvey, 1995.

Goldstein, William. "Books on Pregnancy, Childbirth, and Childrearing: A Checklist." *Publishers Weekly* 223 (22 April 22 1983): 34–41.

Goodell, William. "Some Ancient Methods of Delivery." *American Journal of Obstetrics* 4 (1872): 663.

————. *A Sketch in the Life and Writings of Luoyse Bourgeois.* Philadelphia, Pa.: Collis, 1876.

Goodlin, Robert C. "Postpartum Vulvar Edema Associated with the Birthing Chair." *American Journal of Obstetrics and Gynecology* 146 (1983): 334.

Goodman, Adrianne. "Maternity Wards Come to Life with Rising Birthrate." *The Los Angles Times,* 21 January 1985, Metro, Part 2, 1.

Gould, Stephen Jay. *The Panda's Thumb: More Reflections in Natural History.* New York: Norton, 1980.

Greene, Melissa. "Latest in Rural Delivery: Natural Childbirth Centers." *Blair and Ketchum's Country Journal* 10 (1983): 34–39.

Gubalke, Wolfgang. *Die Hebamme im Wandel der Zeiten: ein Beitrag zur Geschichte des Hebammenwesens.* Hannover, Germany: Staude, 1985.

Guillemeau, Jean. *Childbirth, or, the Happy Delivery of Women.* London: A. Hatfield, 1612.

Guillemin, Jeanne Harley. "The Business of Childbirth." *Society* 23 (1986): 48–54.

Haberling, Elseluise. *Beiträge zur Geschichte des Hebammenstandes.* Berlin: Elwin Staube, 1940.

Haberling, W. *German Medicine.* New York: P. B. Hoeber, Inc., 1934.

Haggard, Howard. *Devils, Drugs, and Doctors.* New York: Pocket Books, 1929.

Haire, Doris. *The Cultural Warping of Childbirth.* Hillsboro, Wash.: International Childbirth Association, 1972.

Hanawalt, Barbara A. "Conception through Infancy in Medieval English Historical and Folklore Sources." *Folklore Forum* 13 (1980): 127–157.

Hand, Wayland D., ed. *American Folk Medicine: A Symposium.* Berkeley: University of California Press, 1976.

Harrar, James Aitken. *The Story of the Lying-In Hospital of the City of New York.* New York: The Society of the Lying-In Hospital, 1938.

Haukeland, Ingvar. "An Alternative Delivery Position: New Delivery Chair Developed and Tested at Köngsberg Hospital." *American Journal of Obstetrics and Gynecology* 141 (1981): 115–117.

Heister, Lorenz. *Chirurgir, in welcher, alles, was zur Wundarzney gehoret, nach der neuesten und besten Art, grundlich abehandelt, und in acht und dreyssi Kupfertafeln die neuerfundene und dienlichste Instrumente, nebst den bequemsten Handriffrn der chirurgischen Operationen und Bandagen deutlich.* Nürnberg, Germany: G. N. Raspe, 1763.

———. *Institution de Chirurgie, ou l'on traite dans un ordre clair et nouveau de tout ce qui a rapport a cet art.* Avignon, France: J. J. Niel, 1770.

Hellman, Alfred Myer. *A Collection of Early Obstetrical Books: An Historical Essay with Bibliographical Descriptions of 37 Items, Including 25 Editions of Roesslin's Rosengarten.* New Haven, Conn.: Alfred Myer Hellman, 1952.

Hellman, Louis M., and Jack A. Pritchard, eds. *Williams Obstetrics.* 14th ed. New York: Appleton-Century-Croft, 1971.

Hodder, Ian. *The Meaning of Things: Material Culture and Symbolic Expression.* London: Urwin Hyman, 1989.

Hoffert, Sylvia. *Private Matters: American Attitudes toward Childbearing and Infant Nurture in the Urban North, 1800–1860.* Urbana: University of Illinois Press, 1989.

Holmes, R. W. "The Fads and Fancies of Obstetrics." *American Journal of Obstetrics and Gynecology* 2 (1921): 22–37.

Hope, Robert Charles. *The Legendary Lore of the Holy Wells of England.* London: Elliot Stock, 1893.

Horenburgin, Anna Elisabeth. *Wohlmeynender und Nötiger Unterricht der Hebammen etc.* Hannover, Germany: Wolflen-Büttel, 1700.

Horten, Jacqueline A., ed. *The Women's Health Data Book: A Profile of Women's Health in the United States.* New York: Elsevier, 1992.

Hosford, Elizabeth. "The Home Birth Movement." *Journal of Nurse-Midwifery* 21 (1976): 15–19.

Householder, Martha. "A Historical Perspective on the Obstetrics Chair." *Surgical Gynecology and Obstetrics* 139 (1974): 423–430.

Howard, Forrest. "Delivery in the Physiologic Position." *Obstetrics and Gynecology* 11 (1958): 318–322.

————. "The Physiologic Position for Delivery." *American Journal of Obstetrics and Gynecology* 78 (1959): 1141–1143.

Hufford, David. "Contemporary Folk Medicine." In *Other Healers: Unorthodox Medicine in America,* edited by Norman Gevitz, 228–264. Baltimore, Md.: Johns Hopkins University Press, 1988.

Hurd-Mead, K. C. *History of Women in Medicine: From the Earliest Times to the Beginning of the 19th Century.* Haddam, Conn.: The Haddam Press, 1938.

Ingerslev, E. "Rösslin's 'Rosegarten': Its Relation to the Past (the Muscio Manuscripts and Soranus) Particularly with Regard to Podalis Version." *Journal of Obstetrics and Gynecology of the British Empire* 15 (1909): 1–92.

Jarcho, Julius. *Postures and Practices during Labor among Primitive People.* New York: Paul B. Hoeber, Inc., 1934.

Jones, Carl. *Alternative Birth, The Complete Guide: Healthy Options for You and Your Baby.* Los Angeles: Jeremy P. Tarcher, Inc., 1991.

Jonson, Ben. *The Magnetic Lady, or, Humors Reconciled.* New York: H. Holt, 1914.

Jordan, Brigitte. "The Hut and the Hospital: Information, Power, and Symbolism in the Artifact of Birth." *Birth and Family Journal* 14 (1987): 36–40.

————. *Birth in Four Cultures. A Crosscultural Investigation of Childbirth in Yucatan, Holland, Sweden, and the United States.* Prospect Heights, Ill.: Waveland Press, 1993.

Jordan, Brigitte, and Sheila Romalis. *Studying Childbirth: The Experience and Methods of a Woman Anthropologist.* Austin: University of Texas Press, 1981.

Kaplan, Gisela T. *Contemporary Western European Feminism.* North Sydney, New South Wales: Allen & Unwin, 1992.

Karlsen, Carol. *The Devil in the Shape of a Woman.* New York: Norton, 1987.

Karmel, Marjorie. *Thank You, Dr. Lamaze.* New York: J. B. Lippincott Co., 1965.

Kay, Margarita. *Anthropology of Human Birth.* Philadelphia, Pa.: F. A. Davis Co., 1982.

Kealey, Linda, ed. *A Not So Unreasonable Claim: Women and Reform in Canada, 1880s–1920s.* Toronto: The Women's Press, 1979.

Kesby, Olivia. "A Case for the Birthing Chair." *Nursing Mirror* 155 (1982): 37.

Kett, Joseph. *The Formation of the American Medical Profession: The Role of Institutions, 1780–1860.* New Haven, Conn.: Yale University Press, 1968.

Kevill-Davies, Sally. *Yesterday's Children.* New York: Antique Collectors' Club, Ltd., 1992.

Kieckhefer, Richard. *European Witch Trails: Their Foundation in Popular and Learned Culture, 1300–1600.* Los Angeles: University of California Press, 1976.

Kilchenstein, Mary Isabelle. "Extremes of the Contemporary Frontier." In *Utopias: The American Experience,* edited by Gairdner B. Moment and Otto F. Kraushaar, 153–178. Metuchen, N.J.: The Scarecrow Press, 1980.

Kilmer, Anne. "The Brick of Birth." *Journal of Near Eastern Studies* 46 (1987): 211–213.

King, A. F. A. "The Physiological Argument in Obstetrical Studies and Practice." *American Journal of Women and Children* 21 (1888): 372.

―――. "Significance of Posture in Obstetrics." *Society of the Lying-In Hospital Bulletin* 5 (1909): 202–212.

King, H. D. "The Evolution of the Male Midwife, Some Remarks on the Obstetrical Literature of Other Ages." *American Journal of Obstetrics* 77 (1918): 177–186.

Klapper, R. J. "The Midwife in Europe." *Nursing Times* 69 (3 May 1973): 586–587.

Kleinman, Arthur. *Patients and Healers in the Context of Culture: An Exploration of the Borderland between Anthropology, Medicine, and Psychiatry.* Berkeley: University of California Press, 1980.

Knauth, Donna. "Effect of Pushing Techniques in Birthing Chair on Length of Second Stage Labor." *Nursing Research* 35 (1986): 49–51.

Knecht, Wagen, ed. *Mrs. Fanny Appleton Longfellow (1817–1861).* New York: Longmans, Green, 1956.

Kosmark, George. "The Favorable and Unfavorable Results of the Practice of Modern Obstetrical Trends and Procedures." *Mississippi Doctor* 16 (1938): 1–11.

Kotulak, Ronald. "A New Stand on Birth, Its Actual Very Ancient Logic: Upright Birth Can Help Ease the Travail." *Chicago Tribune,* 16 August 1987, Tempo.

Kreppel, Marie Curro. "Books I've Read: Crosscurrents in Obstetrics and Literary Childbirth." *Atlantis: A Women's Studies Journal* 10 (1984): 1–11.

Kuntner, Liselotte. *Die Gebärhaltung der Frau: Schwangerschaft und Geburt aus geschichtlicher, völkerkundlicher und medizinischer Sict.* München, Germany: Marseille Verlag, 1985.

Kunzle, David. *Fashion and Fetishism: A Social History of the Corset, Tight-Lacing, and Forms of Body-Sculpture in the West.* Totowa, N.J.: Rowman & Littlefield, 1982.

Lake, A. "Childbirth in America: A National Scandal." *McCalls,* January 1976, 83.

Leap, N., and B. Hunter. *The Midwife's Tale: An Oral History of Childbirth in the Twentieth Century.* London: Scarlet Press, 1993.

Leavitt, Judith Walzer. "Down to Death's Door." In *Proceedings of the Second Motherhood Symposium: Childbirth,* edited by Sophie Colleau, 113–136. Madison: University of Wisconsin Press, 1982.

―――. "Science Enters the Birthing Room: Obstetrics in America Since the Eighteenth Century." *The Journal of American History* 70 (1983): 281–304.

―――. "Birthing and Anesthesia: The Debate over the Twilight Sleep." In *Women and Health in America,* edited by Judith Walzer Leavitt, 175–184. Madison: University of Wisconsin Press, 1984.

————. *Brought to Bed: Childbearing in America, 1750 to 1950.* New York: Oxford University Press, 1986.

Leavitt, Judith Walzer, ed. *Women and Health in America.* Madison: The University of Wisconsin Press, 1984.

Leavitt, Judith Walzer, and Ronald L. Numbers, eds. *Sickness and Health in America: Readings in the History of Medicine and Public Health.* Madison: University of Wisconsin Press, 1985.

Lerman, Alice. *Birth Environments: Emerging Trends and Implications for Design.* Milwaukee: University of Wisconsin Press, 1991.

Lerner, Gerda. "The Lady and the Mill Girl: Changes in the Status of Women in the Age of Jackson." *American Studies Journal* 10 (1969): 5–15.

————. *The Majority Finds Its Past: Placing Women in History.* New York: Oxford University Press, 1979.

Levack, Brian P. *The Witch-Hunt in Early Modern Europe.* London: Longman, 1987.

————. *Witchcraft, Women, and Society.* New York: Garland, 1992.

Lewis, Jan. "'Sally Has Been Sick': Pregnancy and Family Limitation among Virginia Gentry Women, 1780–1830." *Journal of Social History* 22 (1988): 5–19.

Lewis, Judith Schneid. *In the Family Way: Childbearing in the British Aristocracy, 1760–1860.* New Brunswick, N.J.: Rutgers University Press, 1986.

Liddell, H. S. "The Birthing Chair in Second Stage Labor." *Australian and New Zealand Journal of Obstetrics and Gynecology* 25 (1985): 65–68.

Litoff, Judy Barrett. *American Midwives, 1860 to the Present.* Westport, Conn.: Greenwood Press, 1978.

————. "The Midwife throughout History." *Journal of Nurse-Midwifery* 27 (1982): 3–11.

————. *The American Midwife Debate: A Sourcebook on Its Modern Origins.* Westport, Conn.: Greenwood Press, 1986.

Lockridge, Kenneth. *Literacy in Colonial New England: An Inquiry into the Social Context of Literacy in the Early Modern West.* New York: W. W. Norton, 1974.

Lubic, Ruth. "Barriers and Conflict in Maternity Care Innovation." Ed.D. diss., Columbia University Teachers College, 1980.

MacDorman, M., and G. Singh. "Midwifery Care, Social and Medical Risk Factors and Birth Outcomes in the U.S.A." *Journal of Epidemiology and Community Health* 52 (1998): 310–317.

MacNab, Elizabeth. *A Legal History of Health Professions in Ontario.* Toronto: Queen's Printer, 1979.

MacPike, Loralee. "The Fallen Women's Sexuality: Childbirth and Censure." *Tennessee Studies in Literature* 27 (1984): 54–71.

Marcus, J. H. "Childbirth and Its Ancient Customs." *New York Medical Journal* 106 (1917): 1213.

Markoe, James. "A Revival of the Obstetrics Chair." *Society of the Lying-In Hospital Bulletin* 9 (1914): 296–306.

————. "Practical Experience with the Obstetrics Chair." *Society of the Lying-In Hospital Bulletin* 10 (1915): 95–101.

Marland, Hilary, ed. *Medicine and Society in Wakefield and Huddersfield, 1780–1870.* Cambridge History of Medicine. Cambridge, U.K.: Cambridge University Press, 1987.

————. *The Art of Midwifery: Early Modern Midwives in Europe.* London: Routledge, 1993.

Marshall, R. "Birth as a Profession." *Nursing Mirror* 156 (1983): 57.

Martin, Emily. *The Woman in the Body: A Cultural Analysis of Reproduction.* Boston: Beacon Press, 1987.

Mathews, Washington. "Myths of Gestation and Parturition." *American Anthropologist* 4 (1902): 737–742.

Mauriceau, Francios. *The Diseases of Women with Child,* translated by Hugh Chamberlain. London: John Darby, 1683.

————. *Observations sur la grossesse et l'accouchement des femmes et sur leurs maladies et celles des enfants nouveaux-nés.* Paris: L'Auteur, 1694.

McCool, William, and Sandi McCool. "Feminism and Nurse-Midwifery." *Journal of Nurse-Midwifery* 34 (1989): 323–334.

McCormack, Patricia. "Birthing Chair Shortens Second Stage of Labor." *United Press International,* 19 October 1981, PM Cycle.

McCormick, Carol P., ed. *Ethnography of Fertility and Birth.* Prospect Heights, Ill.: Waveland Press, 1994.

McDowell, Edwin. "Books Are Proliferating on the Care of Children." *New York Times,* 29 August 1984, Section C, 1.

McKibben, Gordon. "Medical Equipment Finds New Life." *The Boston Globe,* 28 December 1989, Economy, 47.

McMaster, G. T. "Ancient Greece, the First Woman Practitioner (Agnodice) of Midwifery and the Care of Infants in Athens, 300 BC." *American Medical* 8 (1912): 202–205.

McMillen, Sally S. *Motherhood in the Old South: Pregnancy, Childbirth, and Infant Rearing.* Baton Rouge: Louisiana State University Press, 1990.

McSwain, Dianne. "Social Networks and Natural Childbirth." Ph.D. diss., Department of Anthropology, University of California, Davis, 1980.

Meckel, Richard A. *"Save the Babies": American Public Health Reform and the Prevention of Infant Mortality, 1850–1929.* Baltimore, Md.: Johns Hopkins University Press, 1990.

Meigs, Charles D. *A Complete Treatise on Midwifery and the Theory and Practice Tokology: Including the Diseases of Pregnancy, Labor, and the Puerperal State.* Philadelphia, Pa.: Lindsay & Blakiston, 1852.

Meiners, Uwe, ed. *Korsetts und Nylonstrümpfe: Frauenunterwäshe als Spiegel von Mode und Gesellschaft Zwischen 1890 und 1960.* Oldenberg, Germany: Isensee Verlag, 1994.

Méndez-Bauer, C., et al. "Effects of Standing Position on Spontaneous Uterine Contractility and Other Aspects of Labor." *Journal of Perinatal Medicine* 3 (1975): 89–100.

Mengert, William. "The Origin of the Male Midwife." *Annals of Medical History* 4 (1932): 453–465.

Mesnard, Jacques. *Les guide des accoucheurs, ou le maistre dans l'art d'accoucher les femmes, et de les soulager sans les maladies & accidens dont elles sont tres souvent attaquees. Ouvrage des plus utiles pour les personnes qui veulent faire une pratique particuliere de l'operation des accoucheurs.* Paris: Chez De Bure, Le Breton, Durand, 1753.

Michaelson, Karen. *Childbirth in America: Anthropological Perspectives.* New York: Bergin & Garvey, 1988.

Mines, Cynthia. "Birthing Rooms Become Featured Attractions to Grab Market Share." *Wichita Business Journal* 3 (1988): 13.

Mitchell, S. Weir. *Doctor and Patient.* 2d ed. Philadelphia, Pa.: J. B. Lippincott & Co., 1888.

Mitchinson, Wendy. "Historical Attitudes toward Women and Childbirth." *Atlantis* 2 (1979): 13–34.

Mitford, Jessica. *The American Way of Birth.* New York: Dutton, 1992.

Morants, Regina. "Professionalism, Feminism, and Gender Role." *Journal of American History* 67 (1980): 568–588.

Mulcahy, Joanne Burke. "'Knowing Women': Narratives of Healing and Traditional Life from Kodiak Island, Alaska." Ph.D. diss., Department of Folklore and Folklife, University of Pennsylvania, 1988.

Muller, Charlotte Feldman. *Health Care and Gender.* New York: Russell Sage Foundation, 1990.

Murphee, A. "A Functional Analysis of Southern Folk Beliefs Concerning Birth." *American Journal of Obstetrics and Gynecology* 102 (1968): 125–134.

Murphy, Edward William. *Lectures on the Principles and Practices of Midwifery.* 2d ed. London: Walton and Maberly, 1862.

Myerhoff, Barbara, and W. Larsen. "The Doctor as Culture Hero: The Rountinization of Charisma." *Human Organization* 24 (1965): 188–193.

Nagai, Hiroshi. "The Management of Labor with a Modern Birthing Chair and Telemetry." Paper presented at the 10th World Congress of Gynecology and Obstetrics, Los Angeles, 17–22 October 1982.

Nash, Charles E. *The History of Augusta: First Settlement and Early Days as a Town, Including the Diary of Mrs. Martha Moore Ballard (1785–1812).* Augusta, Maine, 1904.

Nihell, Elizabeth. *A Treatise on the Art of Midwifery Setting Forth Various Abuses Therein, Especially as to the Practice with Instruments: The Whole Serving to Put All Rational Inquirers in a Fair Way of Very Safely Forming Their Own Judgment upon the Question, Which Is Left to Employ in Cases of Pregnancy and Lying-In A Man-Midwife or, a Midwife.* London: A. Manly, 1760.

Oakley, Ann. *Women Confined: Toward a Sociology of Childbirth.* New York: Schocken Books, 1980.

―――. *The Captured Womb: A History of the Medical Care of Pregnant Women.* Oxford: Basil Blackwell Ltd., 1984.

―――. *Helpers in Childbirth: Midwifery Today.* New York: Hemisphere Publication Corp., 1990.

O'Dowd, Michael J., and Elliot E. Philipp. *The History of Obstetrics and Gynaecology.* New York: Parthenon Publishing Group, 1994.

Oppenheimer, Jo. "Childbirth in Ontario: The Transition from Home to Hospital in the Early Twentieth Century." In *Delivering Motherhood: Maternal Ideologies and Practices in the 19th and 20th Centuries,* edited by Katherine Arnup, Andrée Lévesque, and Ruth Roach Pierson, 61–62. New York: Routledge, 1990.

Ortiz, T. "From Hegemony to Subordination: Midwives in Early-Modern Spain." In *The Art of Midwifery: Early Modern Midwives in Europe,* edited by H. Marland, 95–114. London: Routledge, 1993.

Osherson, Samuel, and Johanna Singhorn. "The Machine Metaphor in Medicine." In *Social Contexts of Health, Illness, and Patient Care,* edited by Elliot Mishler, 218–249. Cambridge, U.K.: Cambridge University Press, 1981.

Osiander, Friedreich Benjamin. *Kurze Nachricht von der Entstehung und Einrichtung der Gesellschaft von Freunden der Entbindungskunst.* Göttingen, Germany, 1795.

―――. *Osiander's Geburtsstelle.* Frankfurt, Germany, 1821.

―――. *Handbuch der Entbindungkunst.* Tübingen, Germany, 1825.

Osiander, Johann Friedrich. *Gemeinsame Deutsche Zeitschrift für Geburtskunde.* Weimar, Germany, 1829.

―――. *Zur Praxis der Geburtshulfe; Beobachtungen und Bemerkungen aus der academischen Entbindungsanstalt zu Gottingen, wahrend der beiden Jahre 1822 und 1832.* Hannover, Germany: Helwing, 1837.

Otten, Carl. "Rebirth of the Birthing Chair." *The Saturday Evening Post,* January/February (1982): 22–24.

Otten, Charlotte F. *English Women's Voices, 1540–1700.* Miami: Florida International University Press, 1992.

―――. "Women's Prayers in Childbirth in Sixteenth Century England." *Women and Language* 16 (1993): 18–21.

Paige, Karen. *The Politics of Reproductive Ritual.* Berkeley: University of California Press, 1981.

Parachini, Allan. "Hospital Campaigns Aim to Deliver More Babies." *Los Angles Times,* 14 September 1987, Home Edition, View, Part 5, 1.

Paré, Ambroise. *Les Oeuvres d' Ambroise Paré.* 1664. Reprint. Lyon, France: Jean Gregoire, 1821.

―――. *On Monsters and Marvels.* 1561. Reprint. Chicago, Ill.: University of Chicago Press, 1982.

Parker, Gail. *The Oven-Birds: American Women on Womanhood, 1820–1920.* Garden City, N.Y.: Doubleday/Anchor, 1972.

Peterson, Karen J. "Technology as the Last Resort in Home Births: The Work of Lay Midwives." *Social Problems* 30 (1983): 272–283.

Pike, Martha, and Janice Grey Armstrong, eds. *A Time to Mourn: Expressions of Grief in American Art.* Stonybrook, N.Y.: The Museum at Stonybrook, 1980.

Pinto, Lucille B. "The Folk Practice of Gynecology and Obstetrics in the Middle Ages." *Bulletin of the History of Medicine* 47 (1973): 513–522.

Ploss, Hermann Heinrich. *Woman: An Historical, Gynecological and Anthropological Compendium.* London: W. Heinemann, Ltd., 1935.

Poovey, Mary. "'Scenes of an Indelicate Nature': The Medical Treatment of Victorian Women." In *The Making of the Modern Body: Sexuality and Society in the Nineteenth Century,* edited by Catherine Gallagher and Thomas Laquer, 37–168. Berkeley: University of California Press, 1987.

———. *Uneven Developments: The Ideological Work of Gender in Mid-Victorian England.* Women in Culture and Society. Chicago, Ill.: University of Chicago Press, 1988.

Power, Sir D'Arcy. *The Birth of Mankind or the Woman's Book: A Bibliographic Study.* London: The Bibliographic Society, 1927.

Prown, Jules David. "Mind in Matter: An Introduction to Material Culture Theory and Method." In *Material Life in American, 1600–1860,* edited by Robert St. George, 17–38. Boston: Northeastern University Press, 1988.

Putnam, Emily. *The Lady: Studies of Certain Significant Phases of Her History.* New York: Sturgis & Walton Co., 1910.

Quinlin, Maurice. *Victorian Prelude: A History of English Manners, 1700–1830.* New York: Columbia University Press, 1941.

Radcliffe, Walter. *Milestones in Midwifery.* Bristol: John Wright & Sons, Ltd., 1967.

Ramazzini, Bernardino. *De Morbis Artificum.* 1713. Reprint. New York: Classics of Medicine Library, 1983.

Raynalde, Thomas. *The Birth of Mankinde; Otherwise Named, the Woman's Booke. Set Forth in English by Thomas Raynalde, Physician and by Him Corrected and Augmented.* London, 1540.

———. *The Byrth of Mankynde, Otherwyse Named the Woman's Booke, Newly Set Forth, Corrected & Augmented, Whole Contents Ye Maye Rede in the Table of the Booke, & Most Playnly in the Prologue by Thomas Raynold, Physician.* London, 1545.

Rigby, Edward. "What Is the Natural Position of a Woman during Labor?" *Medical Times and Gazette* 36 (3 October 1857): 345–346.

Riska, Elianne. *Power, Politics, and Health: Forces Shaping American Medicine.* Helsinki: Finnish Society of Sciences and Letters, 1985.

Robb, Hunter. "The Writings of L. Bourgeois." *Bulletin of the Johns Hopkins Hospital* 4 (1893): 75–81.

———. "The Works of Justine Siegemundin, The Midwife." *Bulletin of the Johns Hopkins Hospital* 5 (1894): 4–13.

———. "The Writings of Marticeau." *Bulletin of the Johns Hopkins Hospital* 6 (1895): 51–57.

Roberts, Helen, ed. *Women, Health and Reproduction.* London: Routledge & Kegan Paul, 1981.

Roberts, Joyce. "Alternative Positions for Childbirth. Part I: First Stage of Labor." *Journal of Nurse-Midwifery* 25 (1980): 11–18.

———. "Alternative Positions for Childbirth. Part II: Second Stage of Labor." *Journal of Nurse-Midwifery* 25 (1980): 13–19.

Romalis, Sheila, and Brigitte Jordan. *Childbirth: Alternatives to Medical Control.* Austin: University of Texas Press, 1981.

Romond, Janis Loomis, and Irene Taylor Baker. "Squatting in Childbirth: A New Look at an Old Tradition." *Journal of Obstetric, Gynecologic and Neonatal Nursing* 14 (1985): 406–411.

Rongy, A. J. *Childbirth Yesterday and Today: The Story of Childbirth through the Ages to the Present.* New York: Emerson Books, 1937.

Rooks, Judith P. "The Context of Nurse-Midwifery in the 1980s: Our Relationships with Medicine, Nursing, Lay-Midwives, Consumers and Health Care Economist." *Journal of Nurse-Midwifery* 28 (1983): 3–8.

———. *Midwifery and Childbirth in America.* Philadelphia, Pa.: Temple University Press, 1997.

Rooks, Judith P., Norman L. Weatherby, Eunice K. M. Ernst, Susan Stapleton, David Rosen, and Allan Rosenfield. "Outcomes of Care in Birth Centers." *New England Journal of Medicine* 321 (1989): 1804–1811.

Rosen, George. *Fees and Fee Bills: Some Economic Aspects of Medical Practice in Nineteenth-Century America.* Baltimore, Md.: Johns Hopkins University Press, 1946.

Rosenberg, Charles E. "The Therapeutic Revolution: Medicine, Meaning, and Social Changes in Nineteenth-Century America." In *The Therapeutic Revolution: Essays in the Social History of Medicine,* edited by Morris Vogel and Charles Rosenberg, 3–25. Philadelphia: University of Pennsylvania Press, 1979.

———. *The Care of Strangers: The Rise of America's Hospital System.* New York: Basic Books, 1987.

Rösslin, Eucharius. *Der Swangern frauen und Hebammen Rosengarten.* Argentine, Germany: Martinus Flach Junior, 1513.

———. [Eucharius Rhodion]. *De Tartu Hominis.* Frankfurt, 1532.

———. *The Birth of Mankinde: Otherwyse Named the Woman's Booke.* London: R. Watkins, 1598.

———. *Eucharius Rösslin's 'Rosengarten' b. gedruckt im jahre 1513,* edited by Gustav Klein. München, Germany: C. Kuhn, 1910.

———. *When Midwifery Became the Male Physician's Province, The Sixteenth Century Handbook: The Rose Garden for Pregnant Women and Midwives. Newly Englished.* Jefferson, N.C.: McFarland & Co., 1994.

Rothman, Barbara Katz. "Anatomy of a Compromise: Nurse-Midwifery and the Rise of the Birth Center." *Journal of Nurse-Midwifery* 28 (1983): 3–7.

———. "Childbirth Management and Medical Monopoly: Midwifery as (Almost) a Profession." *Journal of Nurse-Midwifery* 29 (1984): 300–306.

———. "Your Pregnancy: New Tests, New Fears." *Glamour* September 1993, 273–275, 312–314.

Rothstein, William G. *The American Physician in the Nineteenth Century: From Sect to Science.* Baltimore, Md.: Johns Hopkins University Press, 1972.

Rueff, Jakob. *Ein schon lustig Trostbuchle in von den Empfangnissen und Geburten der Menschen.* Zurich, 1544.

————. *du Conceptu et generatione hominis.* Tiguri, Switzerland: Christophorus Froschoverus, 1554.

————. *Hebammen Buch, darus man alle Heimligkeit desz weiblichen Geschlechts erlehrnen, welcherlev Gestalt der Mensch in Mütter Leib empfangen, zunimpt und geboren wirdt.* Frankfurt, 1580.

————. *The Expert Midwife.* London: Griffin, 1637.

————. *Ein schön lustig Trostbuchle von den Empfengknuben und Geburten der Menschen.* Zurich: Bibliophile Drucke, 1981.

Rutenberg, Sharon. "Birthing Seat Is Said to Ease Mother through Childbearing." *United Press International,* 2 August 1983, Lifestyles.

Ruzek, Sheryl Bert. *The Women's Health Movement.* New York: Praeger, 1978.

Sacks, Elizabeth. *Shakespeare's Images of Pregnancy.* New York: St. Martin's Press, 1980.

Sandelowski, Margaret. *Pain, Pleasure, and American Childbirth: From the Twilight Sleep to the Read Method, 1914–1960.* Westport, Conn.: Greenwood Press, 1984.

Savonarola, Giovanni. *Practica major,* edited by Joannis Michaelis Savonarola. Venice: Apud Vincentium Valgrisium, 1560.

Scheffey, Lewis C. "The Early History and the Transition Period of Obstetrics and Gynecology in Philadelphia." *Annals of Medical History* 2 (1940): 215–216.

Schlereth, Thomas J. *Material Culture Studies in America.* Nashville, Tenn.: American Association for State and Local History, 1982.

Schmidtmüller, Johann Anton. *Handbuch der medizinischen Geburtshulfe zur Grundlage bei akademischen Vorlesungen.* Frankfurt: Andrea, 1809.

Schmitz, Britta. *Hebammen in Munster: historische Entwicklung, Lebens-und Arbeitsumfeld, berufliches Selbstverstandnis.* Munster, Germany: Waxmann, 1994.

Schnucker, R. V. "Pregnancy, Delivery, and the English Puritans." *History of Childhood Quarterly* 1 (1974): 637–658.

Scholten, Catherine. "On the Importance of the Obstetrik Art: Changing Customs of Childbirth in America." *William and Mary Quarterly* 34 (1977): 434–438.

————. *Childbearing in American Society, 1650–1850.* New York: New York University Press, 1985.

Schrader, Catharina Gertruida. *Mother and Child Were Saved: The Memoirs (1693–1740) of the Frisian Midwife Catharina Schrader.* Amsterdam: Rodopi, 1987.

Schumann, E. A. "The Deities Concerned with Childbirth among Ancient Peoples." *American Journal of Obstetrics and Gynecology* 10 (1925): 576.

Schurz, A. R. "Erfahrungen mit dem E K-Entbindungsstuhl." *Geburtsh. u. Frauenheilk* 41 (1981): 868–870.

Schweighäuser, J. F. *Aufsätze über einige physiologische und Praktische Gegenstände der Geburtshuelfe.* Nürnberg, Germany, 1817.

Sermon, William. *The Ladies Companion, or, The English Midwife Wherein Is Demonstrated the Manner and Order How Women Ought to Govern Themselves during the Whole Time of Their Breeding Children and of Their Difficult Labour, Hard Travail and Lying-In.* London: Edward Thomas, 1671.

Sewell, Jane Elliot. *Cesarean Section<m>A Brief History: A Brochure to Accompany an Exhibition on the History of Cesarean Section at the National Library of Medicine. 30 April 1993–31 August 1993.* Washington, D.C.: American College of Obstetricians and Gynecologists, 1993.

Shannahan, Mary Davies, and Barbara Hansen Cottrell. "Effect of the Birth Chair on Duration of Second Stage Labor, Fetal Outcome, and Maternal Blood Loss." *Nursing Research* 34 (1985): 89–92.

———. "The Effects of Birth Chair Delivery on Maternal Perceptions." *Journal of Obstetrics and Gynecologic and Neonatal Nursing* 18 (1989): 323–326.

Sharp, Jane. *The Midwives Book, or Whole Art of Midwifery: Directing Childbearing Women How to Behave.* London, 1671.

Shorter, Edward. *A History of Women's Bodies.* New York: Basic Books, 1982.

———. *Women's Bodies: A Social History of Women's Encounter with Health, Ill-Health, and Medicine.* New York: Transaction Publishers, 1991.

Shryock, Richard. *Public Relations of the Medical Profession in Great Britain and the United States, 1600–1870.* New York: P. B. Hueber, 1930.

———. *The Development of Modern Medicine: An Interpretation of the Social and Scientific Factors Involved.* 1936. Reprint. Madison: University of Wisconsin Press, 1979.

Shultz, Gladys. "Cruelty in Maternity Wards." *Ladies Home Journal* 75 (May 1958): 35–39.

———. "Journal Mothers Report on Cruelty in Maternity Ward." *Ladies Home Journal* 75 (August 1958): 44–45, 55–61.

Siebold, Adam Elias von. "Kritik einiger Geburtszangen nebst Beschreibung, Abbildung und Kritik der von ihm verbesserten Geburtszange." *Lucina* 1 (1802): 206–224.

———. *Ubhandlung über den neuen von ihm erfunden Geburtstuhl.* Weimar, Germany: Berlage des Landes, 1804.

———. *Über ein bequemes und einfaches Kissen zur Erleichterung des Geburt und Geburtshilfe.* Berlin, 1819.

Siebold, E. C. J. von. *Versuch einer der Geburtshülfe.* Berlin: Enslin, 1839.

Siegemundin, Justine. *Die Chur-Brandenburgische Hoff Wehe-Mütter.* Colin an der Spree, Germany: Ulrich Liebperten, 1690.

Siennik, Marcin. *Herbarz.* Krakow: W Druk. Mikolaia Szarfenberga, 1568.

Simon, Francesca. "Childbirth through the Ages." *Parents* 58 (1983): 82–177.

Smellie, William A. *A Collection of Cases and Observations in Midwifery to Illustrate His Former Treatise, or First Volume, on That Subject.* London: D. Wilson and T. Dorcham, 1758.

———. *Treatise on the Theory and Practice of Midwifery.* London: D. Wilson, 1779.

————. *Treatise on the Theory and Practice of Midwifery,* edited by Alfred McClintock. London: The New Sydenham Society, 1876.

Smith, Antony. *The Body.* New York: Walker & Co., 1968.

Smith, W. Tyler. "Obstetrics as a Profession." *Lancet* 2 (1847): 451–460.

————. "Obstetrics as a Science." *British and Foreign Medico-Chirurgical Review* 4 (1849): 501–510.

Smith-Rosenberg, Carroll. "Puberty to Menopause: The Cycle of Femininity in Nineteenth-Century America." In *Clio's Consciousness Raised,* edited by Mary Hartmen and Lois Banner, 23–37. New York: Harper & Row, 1974.

————. "The Female World of Love and Ritual." *Signs* 1 (1975): 1–29.

Smith-Rosenberg, Carroll, and Charles Rosenberg. "The Female Animal: Medical and Biological Views of Woman and Her Role in Nineteenth-Century America." *Journal of American History* 60 (1973): 332–356.

Speert, Harold. *Iconographia Gyniatrica: A Pictorial History of Gynecology and Obstetrics.* New York: F. A. Davis, 1973.

————. *Obstetrics and Gynecology in America.* Chicago, Ill.: American College of Obstetricians and Gynecologists, 1980.

Spencer, Herbert. *The History of British Midwifery from 1650–1800.* London: John Bale, Sons, and Danielson, Ltd., 1927.

Stark, J. C. *Archiv für Geburtshuelfe, Frauenzimmer und neugebore Kinder Krankheiten.* Jena, Germany: Wolfgang Stahl, 1787–1793.

Starr, Paul. *The Social Transformation of American Medicine.* New York: Basic Books, 1982.

Steidele, Raphael Johann. *Lehrbuch von der Hebammenkunst: mit Kupfern versehen. Dritte verbossorto und vormehrte Auflage.* Vienna: Joh. Thomas Edlen v. Trattnern, 1784

————. *Verhaltensregeln für Schwangere, Gebärende und Kinderbetterinne in der Stadt und auf dem Lande.* Vienna: Johann David Horlingschen Buchhandlung, 1787.

Stein, Georg Wilhelm. *Kurze Beschreibung eines neuen Geburtsstuhls und Bettes.* Kassel, Germany: Henrich Schmiedt, 1772.

Sterne, Lawrence. *The Life and Opinions of Tristram Shandy, Gentleman,* edited by James Aiken Work. Indianapolis, Ind.: The Odyssey Press, 1940.

Stevens, Rosemary. *In Sickness and in Wealth: American Hospitals in the Twentieth Century.* New York: Basic Books, 1989.

Stewart, David. "Notes." *NAPSAC News* Fall (1981): 8.

Stewart, Jacqueline Williamson. "Myths and Beliefs Surrounding Pregnancy and Childbirth." M.A. thesis, California State University, Dominguez Hills, 1980.

Stewart, Peter, Edith Hillan, and Andrew A. Calder. "A Randomized Trail to Evaluate the Use of a Birth Chair for Delivery." *Lancet* 1 (1983): 1296–1298.

St. George, Robert. "'Set Thine House in Order': The Domestication of the Yeomanry in 17th Century New England." In *New England Begins: The Seventeenth Century,* edited by Jonathan Fairbanks and Robert Trent, 165–172. Boston: Museum of Fine Art, 1982.

————. "Artifacts of Regional Consciousness in the Connecticut River Valley,

1700–1780." In *Material Life in America, 1600–1860,* edited by Robert St. George, 335–356. Boston: Northeastern University Press, 1988.

St. George, Robert, ed. *Material Life in America, 1600–1860.* Boston: Northeastern University Press, 1988.

Stucky, Jean Paul. *Der Gebarsthul: Die Grunde für sein Verschwinden im Deutschen Sparachbereich.* Zurich: Juris, 1965.

Sullivan, Deborah A., and Rose Weitz. *Labor Pains: Modern Midwives and Home Birth.* New Haven, Conn.: Yale University Press, 1988.

Susie, Debra Anne. *In the Way of Our Grandmothers: A Cultural View of Twentieth-Century Midwifery in Florida.* Athens: University of Georgia Press, 1988.

Swingley, Pat. "Childbirth Fair a Special Delivery for Parents-to-Be." *The Tennessean,* 31 March 1992, D3.

Tally, Frances Maybell. *From the Mystery of Conception to the Miracle of Birth: An Historical Survey of Beliefs and Rituals Surrounding the Pregnant Women in Germanic Folk Tradition, Including Modern American Folklore.* Los Angeles: University of California Press, 1978.

Tarter, Michele Lise. "Nursing the New Wor(l)d: The Writings of Quaker Women in Early America." *Women & Language* 16 (1993): 22–26.

Tatlock, Lynne. "Speculum Feminarum: Gendered Perspectives on Obstetrics and Gynecology in Early Modern Germany." *Signs* 17 (1992): 725–760.

Taylor, Lloyd C. *The Medical Profession and Social Reform, 1885–1945.* New York: St. Martin's Press, 1974.

Temesváry, Rudolf. *Volksbräuche und Aberglauben in der Geburtshilfe und der Pflege des Neugebornen in Ungarn.* Leipzig, Germany: Th. Grieben's Verlag, 1900.

Thom, Mary. "Dilemmas of the New Birth Technologies." *Ms Magazine* 16 (1988): 70–76.

Thomas, Ian, ed. *Culpepper's Book of Birth.* London: Grange Books, 1993.

Thompson, C. J. S. "The Parturition Chair: Its History and Use." *Proceedings of the Royal Society of Medicine* 15 (1921): 13–20.

Thoms, Herbert. *Chapters in American Obstetrics.* Springfield, Ill.: Charles C. Thomas, 1933.

———. *Our Obstetric Heritage; The Story of Safe Childbirth.* Hamden, Conn.: Shoe String Press, 1960.

Thorwald, Jurgen. *Macht und Geheimnis der fruhen Arzte; Agypten, Babylonien, Indien, China, Mexiko, Peru.* München, Germany: Droemer, Knaur, 1962.

Thronton, Peter. *Seventeenth Century Interior Decoration in England, France and Holland.* New Haven, Conn.: Yale University Press, 1978.

———. *The Furnishings and Decoration of Ham House.* London: Furniture Historical Society, 1980.

Towler, Jean, and Joan Bramall, eds. *Midwives in History and Society.* London: Croom Helm, 1986.

Trent, Robert. "The Wendell Couch." *Maine Antique Digest* 19 (1991): 34–37.

Tröhler, U. *Armamentarium Obstetricum Göttingense: Ein Historische Sammlung zür Geburtsmedizin.* Göttingen, Germany: Vanderhoeck und Ruprecht, 1987.

Trunzo, Candance E. "The New Birthing Options May Be More Congenial than Hospitals—and Less Costly—But They're Also More Risky." *Time* (13 December 1989): 205.

Turner, Ann Warren. *Rituals of Birth: From Prehistory to the Present.* New York: D. McKay Co., 1978.

Ulrich, Laurel Thatcher. *Good Wives: Image and Reality in the Lives of Women in Northern New England, 1650–1750.* New York: Vintage Books, 1980.

———. "The Living Mother of a Living Child: Midwifery and Mortality in Post-Revolutionary New England." *William and Mary Quarterly* 46 (1989): 27–48.

———. *A Midwife's Tale: The Life of Martha Ballard, Based on Her Diary, 1785–1812.* New York: Vintage Books, 1990.

U.S. Preventative Services Task Force. *Guide to Clinical Preventative Services: An Assessment of the Effectiveness of 169 Interventions.* Baltimore, Md.: Williams and Wilkins, 1993.

Valenti, C., et. al. "Birthing in an Upright Position." Paper presented at the LXI Congresso della Societa Italiana di Ginecologiae Ostetricia, Rome, 31 May–2 June 1982.

Van Doren, Mark, ed. *Samuel Sewall's Diary.* New York: Russell & Russell, 1963.

Villerme, L. R. "Siége." In *Dictionnaire,* vol. 51, edited by L. Panckouche, 253–259. Paris, 1821.

Vinay, J. "Hospitals Specialize Services to Attract More Women Patients." *Rocky Mountain Business Journal* 36 (1985): 12–14.

Vogel, Morris. *The Invention of the Modern Hospital, Boston, 1870–1930.* Chicago, Ill.: University of Chicago Press, 1980.

Völter, Christopher. *Neueröffnete Hebammenschule.* Sturtgart, Germany, 1722.

Vrazo, Fawn. "Study Links Mom's Labor to Baby's IQ." *Arizona Daily Star,* 2 May 1991, A2.

Wadsworth, William Scott. "Medicine in the Colonies." Paper read before the Pennsylvania Society of the Order of the Founders and Patriots of America, 14 January 1910.

Wehrli, Ida. *Das Offentliche Medizinalwessen der Stadt Baden im Aau.* Aarau, Switzerland: H. R. Sauerländer & Co., 1927.

Welter, Barbara. "The Cult of True Womanhood, 1820–1860." *American Quarterly* 18 (1966): 151–174.

———. *The Woman Question in American History.* American Problem Studies. Hinsdale, Ill.: Dryden Press, 1973.

———. *Dimity Convictions: The American Woman in the Nineteenth Century.* Athens: Ohio University Press, 1976.

Wertz, Richard, and Dorothy Wertz. *Lying-In: A History of Childbirth in America.* New Haven, Conn.: Yale University Press, 1989.

Wheeler, Eunice. "Alternative Settings for Childbirth: A Comparative Analysis." Ph.D. diss., Department of Sociology, University of North Carolina at Chapel Hill, 1979.

White, Charles. *A Treatise on the Management of Pregnancy and Lying-In Women.* London: Edward and Charles Dilly, 1791.

White, J. W. "Four Thousand Years of Obstetrics." *American Journal of Surgery* 11 (1931): 564–572.

Whitridge, William. "Medical Education and the Midwife Problem in the United States." *Journal of the American Medical Association* 58 (1912): 1–7.

Williams, W. H. *A Concise Treatise on the Progress of Medicine Since the Year 1573.* Ipswich, Suffolk, 1804.

Willis, Evan. *Medical Dominance: The Division of Labour in Australian Health Care.* Sydney: George Allen & Unwin Australia Pty. Ltd., 1983.

―――. *Illness and Social Relations: Issues in the Sociology of Health Care.* St. Leonards, New South Wales: Allen & Unwin, 1994.

Wilson, Adrian. "The Ceremony of Childbirth and Its Interpretations." In *Women as Mothers in Pre-Industrial England: Essays in Memory of Dorothy McLaren,* edited by V. Fildes, 68–107. London: Routledge, 1990.

―――. *The Making of Man-Midwifery: Childbirth in England, 1660–1770.* Cambridge, Mass.: Harvard University Press, 1995.

Witkowsky, G. T. *Histories des Accouchements chez tous les Peuples.* Paris: Steinheil, 1887.

Wolveridge, J. *Speculum Matricis, or the Expert Midwives Handmaid.* London: E. Okes, 1671.

Wood, Anne Douglas. "'The Fashionable Diseases': Woman's Complaints and Their Treatment in Nineteenth-Century America." *Journal of Interdisciplinary History* 4 (1973): 25–52.

World Health Organization. "Appropriate Technology for Birth." *Lancet* 1 (1985): 436–437.

Wright, Louis, and Marion Tingling, eds. *The Secret Diary of William Byrd of Webster, 1709–1792.* Richmond, Ga.: The Dietz Press, 1941.

Wurnig, Peter. "Der Gebärstuhl von Hallstatt Forschungen und Forscher der Tiroler." *Ärzeschule* 2 (1948):50.

Zax, Melvin, Arnold J. Saneroff, and Janet E. Farmer. "Childbirth Education, Maternal Attitudes, and Delivery." *American Journal of Obstetrics and Gynecology* 123 (1975): 185–191.

Zilboorg, Gregory. *The Medical Man and the Witch during the Renaissance.* Baltimore: Johns Hopkins University Press, 1935.

Index